I0485171

Shadows of the Mind

Inside the Minds of the World's Deadliest Serial Killers

By
Jeff A. Schwarz

Copyright 2024 Jeff A. Schwarz. All rights reserved.

No part of this book may be reproduced in any form or by any electronic or mechanical means including information storage and retrieval systems, without permission in writing from the author. The only exception is by a reviewer, who may quote short excerpts in a review.

Although the author and publisher have made every effort to ensure that the information in this book was correct at press time, the author and publisher do not assume and hereby disclaim any liability to any party for any loss, damage, or disruption caused by errors or omissions, whether such errors or omissions result from negligence, accident, or any other cause.

This publication is designed to provide accurate and authoritative information with regard to the subject matter covered. It is sold with the understanding that the publisher is not engaged in rendering professional services. If legal advice or other expert assistance is required, the services of a competent professional should be sought.

The fact that an organization or website is referred to in this work as a citation and/or a potential source of further information does not mean that the author or the publisher endorses the information the organization or website may provide or recommendations it may make.

Please remember that Internet websites listed in this work may have changed or disappeared between when this work was written and when it is read.

Shadows of the Mind

Inside the Minds of the World's Deadliest Serial Killers

Table of Contents

Introduction

Serial killers captivate the collective imagination. They embody an enigma that whispers to our deepest fears and curiosities. They're human, like us, yet they commit acts that defy comprehension, triggering both revulsion and a reluctant intrigue. How does someone become a killer? Can we predict such transformations, or are they unknowable until it's too late? This book seeks to plumb the depths of these questions, navigating through the murky waters of psychology, crime, and justice that define some of history's most notorious killers.

The fascination with serial killers isn't new. Tales of individuals who prey upon society have been recounted for centuries. Yet, the modern era—illuminated by advances in psychology and criminal investigation—offers us new lenses through which we might understand these chilling figures. The 20th century alone is littered with names that strike fear into our hearts: Ted Bundy, Jeffrey Dahmer, and John Wayne Gacy, to name but a few.

In unraveling the threads of their lives, we embark on a journey through their formative years and backgrounds, striving to grasp the early influences that shaped them. Was it genetic predisposition or a tumultuous upbringing that cast the die? Or, perhaps, a sinister combination of both? This book examines the genesis of a killer, scrutinizing their early environments with a rigor that mirrors the investigative processes that first brought them to light.

With each chapter, we aim to not only recount the chilling narratives of infamous figures but to delve into the psychological profiles that accompany their storied crimes. These aren't merely tales of horror, but complex studies of human behavior gone awry. By stepping into the shoes of these individuals, if only for a moment, we may gain insights into the mechanisms of their minds—understanding that, even within the darkest recesses, there exists a twisted logic, a method to the madness.

The role of nature versus nurture is a recurring theme, a thread we pull at repeatedly throughout this exploration. A significant portion of this book is dedicated to understanding how these factors intertwine to produce a serial killer. Do environmental influences sow the seeds of violence, or do hidden genetic codes preordain a descent into darkness? This age-old debate takes on new life as we examine the intricate dance between these two forces, bolstered by advances in psychological and genetic research.

Furthermore, the pursuit of understanding serial killers is not an academic exercise alone. It directly informs the evolving practices of law enforcement and justice systems worldwide, with efforts focused on prevention, capture, and justice. Techniques of evasion employed by these individuals highlight the challenges faced by those tasked with bringing them to justice, while breakthroughs in profiling and investigation offer hope for future prevention.

As media and public perception play substantial roles in shaping our understanding, we must also consider how narratives crafted by journalists and authors contribute to public fascination while sometimes misinforming or sensationalizing. Our coverage extends to these aspects, exploring how they influence both fear and understanding within society.

Ultimately, this book is not just an exploration of criminality but of humanity itself. It compels us to reflect on what lies within us all, on the tenuous boundaries that define societal norms and the aberrations that emerge when those boundaries are transgressed. The exploration of serial killers offers not only a study in deviance but a window into the complex and often contradictory nature of humanity. It's a reminder of both our capacity for evil and our relentless pursuit of understanding and justice.

We invite you into the minds of some of history's most notorious figures—not to glorify their actions but to seek understanding. Through these pages, we endeavor to shine a light into the darkest corners of human behavior, to learn, and perhaps, to find ways to prevent such tragedies in the future. This journey demands an honest and often unsettling exploration of the human psyche, as we attempt to piece together the mosaic of criminal minds and, in turn, the imperfections and aspirations of our justice system. Each entry offers a chapter in a narrative as old as humanity itself—a search for comprehension amid chaos.

Chapter 1:
The Genesis of a Killer

In the dim corners of the human psyche, where shadows blend with reality, the origins of a killer begin to take shape—a collision of circumstance, environment, and an elusive spark that ignites a darker path. Early childhood, often marked by longing for acceptance or a desperate cry for understanding, plays a crucial role in molding these infamous figures. As the world bears witness to their chilling acts, it becomes strikingly clear that the genesis of such individuals lies far beneath the surface, hidden in the echoes of trauma and the whispers of societal neglect. Within the walls of their formative homes, perhaps devoid of warmth or riddled with discord, the scaffolding of their twisted personas is erected. These early influences, often overlooked, are as significant as the notorious deeds that etch their names into history. To dissect the mind of a killer is to peer into a shattered prism, reflecting not just their reality but ours. As we seek to understand, we grapple with the daunting question: are killers born, or are they shaped by the shadows of their past?

Understanding Early Influences

When unraveling the genesis of a killer, it becomes vital to delve deeply into those formative experiences that set the stage for future atrocities. The early years of a person's life are akin to a delicate chute, through which they can either be nurtured safely or dangerously nudged towards aberration. Understanding these early influences offers some clarity into how seemingly ordinary environments can mold extraordinary malevolence.

Many notorious figures who later gained infamy in the realm of serial crimes share not only the chilling headlines they've inspired but also eerily similar backgrounds. Childhood trauma appears to be a recurrent motif in their collective narratives. Abuse, neglect, or the absence of a stable figure can anchor a child in an abyss of instability and begin to fray the edges of their empathy. The shadow of a tormented childhood often looms large, transmuting latent potential for destructiveness into horrifying reality.

Consider the influence of family dynamics, often the first arena where a future killer's worldview is forged. In a household ravaged by dysfunction, a child may internalize chaotic interactions as the norm. Where most might seek stability and love, they find volatility and resentment. This dissonance can lead to a blurring of moral boundaries, a dangerous precursor to criminal behavior. The absence of nurturing can lead them down darker avenues, as they seek to assert control or express buried rage.

Additionally, early exposure to violence, whether witnessed directly or through secondhand accounts, has a profound impact on a child's psyche. The line between fantasy and reality can become dangerously blurred, creating a fertile ground for developing violent tendencies. For some children, violence becomes not just accepted but expected—a tool for expressing emotion or resolving conflict when all others have failed.

With the advent of peer interactions, a child might further assimilate their distorted perceptions shaped at home. The playground and classroom become testing grounds for social beliefs and attitudes. Those who experienced bullying or social isolation may retreat further into themselves, building a cocoon of resentment and fantasies of revenge. The cruel hierarchies formed by peers can exacerbate feelings of inadequacy and drive a young mind towards thoughts of violent reprisal.

In certain cases, a supposed genetic predisposition to violence is exacerbated by these environmental factors. Not every child who experiences trauma or violence becomes a killer, suggesting that inherent biological factors can also play a role. The interaction of environmental stimuli with pre-existing genetic conditions could illuminate some paths that lead to future criminality. Imbalances in brain chemistry or inherited personality disorders may render some individuals more susceptible to incorporating violence into their identities.

The role of media and cultural influences can't be discounted in the shaping of a young mind's understanding of violence. In a society steeped in sensationalism and hyperbole, children exposed to media portrayals of violence may begin to view such actions as glamorous or validating. Serial killers, in particular, have at times been portrayed with an enigmatic allure that can be dangerously enticing for an impressionable mind searching for identity and significance.

In chronicling these insidious influences, the aim is not to absolve responsibility but to comprehend the crucible from which such extreme behaviors arise. Understanding the genesis of a killer requires a nuanced approach, examining how external forces and internal predispositions coalesce to create a mindset capable of unimaginable brutality. It's often in these early encounters with neglect, abuse, and violence that the seeds of future actions are sown, maturing over time into malicious intent.

These experiences form a precarious foundation that psychopaths and sociopaths alike may build upon. Identifying such influences offers a pathway not solely for reflection but for prevention— opportunities to intervene before the untangling threads of psychology and circumstance weave the fabric of a monstrous identity. By shining a light on these murky waters from the past, we arm ourselves with the wisdom to potentially divert others from a path that veers into darkness.

Psychological Profiles of Notoriety

Within the labyrinthine corridors of human nature lies an unsettling truth: some individuals devolve into predators, shaping themselves into the architects of mayhem that society has come to fear. To untangle the minds of these notorious killers, one must begin not with their acts but with their psychological underpinnings. These profiles, marked by complexity, often originate in the depths of early traumas and twisted developmental paths. The raw material of their nature is sculpted by chaotic environments and, sometimes, a genetic tick that manifests in malevolent ways.

Each notorious figure we've turned our lens on possesses a distinct psychological blueprint. These profiles reveal commonalities as well as stark differences. For instance, the charismatic psychopath often relies on charm and manipulation to ensnare victims, leveraging their attributes for malicious ends. In contrast, some may withdraw into isolation, letting their fantasies fester until they burst into horrific acts. Despite differing methods, these killers share an uncanny ability to lead double lives, their true selves hidden beneath a veneer of normalcy.

Consider the case of those with antisocial personality disorders, a common thread in many notorious profiles. This disorder often foreshadows a disregard for social norms, an absence of empathy, and a penchant for deceit. The construct of a moral compass spins wildly in these individuals, often influenced by early experiences of violence or neglect. Embedded within is a propensity for thrill-seeking behavior that escalates over time, spiraling from petty crimes to more sinister ventures.

On the other hand, rage-fueled killers may not share this cold detachment. Instead, their acts of violence are impulsive and uncontrolled, manifestations of deep-seated anger often directed at specific individuals or groups. In these cases, the psychological profile uncovers an intricate web of internal conflicts and unresolved grievances. Such killers might view their acts as justified retribution or even necessary purges of societal wrongs, adding layers of complexity to their psychological studies.

Psychopathy and sociopathy, while often used interchangeably in popular parlance, have clinical distinctions that help demarcate the profiles of different killers. Psychopaths tend to possess a blend of charm and wiliness, their actions meticulous and executed with chilling precision. Meanwhile, sociopaths are more erratic and prone to explosive outbursts, often forming deeper connections with a small group or an individual before eventually turning violent. These nuanced differences inform investigative approaches and psychological evaluations.

Analyzing the family history of these individuals often unravels a cycle of abuse and neglect. Many notorious killers experienced troubled upbringings, marked by inconsistent parenting, exposure to violence, or substance abuse. Such environments stoke the fires of destructive tendencies, reinforcing a belief in their own dominance or worthlessness. In some cases, these killers even witnessed violence firsthand, internalizing brutality as a norm rather than aberration, setting the groundwork for a lifetime of skewed perceptions and violent inclinations.

Moreover, attachment theory offers another prism through which we view these psychological profiles. Disrupted early attachments can lead to the inability to form healthy relational bonds later in life, resulting in affective coldness or intense dependency. While some killers maintain superficial relationships, others experience deep-seated loneliness, nurturing a simmering resentment towards society. This alienation becomes fertile ground for dark fantasies that eventually spill into reality.

It's crucial to consider the role of environmental stressors, too. The social surroundings, characterized by poverty, social isolation, or discrimination, may contribute to the evolution of the killer's psyche. These stressors create a pressure-cooker environment where fantasies of violence become a tantalizing escape from perceived injustices or failures. The interplay between nature and nurture becomes evident here, with genetic predispositions possibly accentuating the effects of a harsh environment.

One must note the presence of delusions or other signs of mental illness in some killers' profiles. Paranoid delusions, auditory hallucinations, and disorganized thinking can obscure the line between reality and the grotesque worlds these individuals construct in their minds. When untreated, these conditions exacerbate tendencies towards violence, making it nearly impossible for the individual to self-regulate or abide by societal laws.

The notorious nature of these killers sometimes lies in their ability to harness their intelligence for twisted plots. Many of them possess above-average intelligence, which they use to skillfully evade capture or manipulate those around them. This aspect of their profiles can be as chilling as their crimes, revealing a premeditated and calculated approach to their heinous acts, which in turn contributes to their enduring infamy.

Conclusively, understanding these psychological profiles involves peeling away the layers that reveal profound disconnection and distorted morality. By examining the elements that coalesce into notoriety, insights are gleaned not only into the minds of these killers but also into the societal structures that allow such minds to develop. Although each profile remains unique, they collectively reflect a warping of human consciousness that obliges examination if we aim to forestall the rise of similar atrocities in future generations.

Thus, the psychological profiles of notoriety are not mere character sketches; they are compasses, pointing both law enforcement and society towards understanding, intervention, and perhaps prevention. Each profile acts as a haunting reminder of what can fester within the human mind when left unchecked or unhealed. As we delve deeper into these profiles, the hope is not only to make sense of the senseless but to trigger meaningful change in how society perceives and treats potential seeds of malevolence before they bloom into horrors.

Chapter 2:
Infamous Killers of the 20th Century

The 20th century saw the unsettling emergence of notorious individuals whose crimes left indelible marks on society, provoking both fear and fascination. From the charming yet deadly Ted Bundy to the methodical butchers like Jeffrey Dahmer, their stories haunt us through the details of their gruesome acts. These killers were not only creatures of darkness but also enigmas that beckoned psychologists and criminologists alike to delve into their fractured psyches. John Wayne Gacy hid sinister secrets beneath his persona of a smiling clown, while the elusive Zodiac Killer taunted investigators with cryptic messages, leaving a trail of mystery that still baffles experts today. Richard Ramirez, with his satanic inclinations, and Albert DeSalvo, named the Boston Strangler, painted chilling portraits of violence. Each name, from Ed Gein to Charles Manson, embodies a chapter of infamy, showcasing uniquely sinister motives and methods. Collectively, these figures challenge our understanding of evil, compelling a continuous exploration of their warped motivations within the annals of crime history. While their actions filled pages of newsprint and television screens, underlying patterns and aberrations provide rare insights into the darker corridors of the human mind, a domain that was previously uncharted to these depths. As we examine their chilling legacies, these infamous killers reveal more than mere acts; they open discussions on the malevolent capacity of human nature.

Ted Bundy

In the shadowy tapestry of the 20th century's most notorious figures, Ted Bundy's name looms large. A killer with both charm and cunning, his story has captivated and horrified generations. Born Theodore Robert Bundy in 1946, he presented himself as the archetype of the all-American boy-next-door. Yet beneath this facade lurked a predatory mind that would claim the lives of at least 30 women across multiple states in the United States.

Bundy's modus operandi was marked by a chilling calculation. He often faked injury, sometimes using a cast or crutch, to lure unsuspecting victims into his car under the guise of needing assistance. This manipulation of trust not only speaks volumes about his intelligence but also about his innate understanding of human nature. It's this ability to exploit empathy and goodwill that makes his crimes all the more unsettling.

The geographic reach of Bundy's crimes was unprecedented, highlighting his meticulous planning and the difficulty law enforcement faced in linking the murders. From Washington to Utah, Oregon to Colorado, his ability to adapt and evade capture stymied investigators for years. It wasn't until his audacious Florida killing spree and subsequent arrest that the full scope of his crimes began to come to light. This cross-country trail of terror underscores the challenges of 20th-century policing, yet also emphasizes Bundy's brazen confidence in navigating state lines.

Psychologically, Bundy presents a fascinating case. Charismatic and articulate, he defied the typical portrait of a serial killer, often engaging with the media and even acting as his own legal defense during trial. This public persona only served to deepen the intrigue surrounding him. Bundy's life and crimes provide fertile ground for exploring the complexities of psychopathy and sociopathy, as he exhibited traits of both, weaving them into a lethal cocktail of deceit and violence.

In the courtroom, Bundy became a media spectacle, turning his trial into a circus of drama and manipulations. His legal proceedings were among the first in the US to be televised, ushering in a new era of public consumption of criminal justice. Even in shackles, Bundy endeavored to control the narrative, demonstrating his exceptional, albeit warped, intelligence.

Ted Bundy's execution in 1989 was met with mixed emotions across the country. Some hailed it as justice served, while others were left haunted by the unanswered questions about why he killed. In looking at Bundy's life, one must wrestle with the enigma he left behind—a man whose heinous acts stand in stark contrast to his self-assured public persona.

Bundy's legacy persists, encapsulating both a morbid curiosity and a profound warning about the interplay of nature, nurture, and the sinister potential of human intellect. His story forces us to confront uncomfortable truths about what lies beneath the masks that individuals can wear. As such, Ted Bundy remains a pivotal figure for those who seek to understand the dark recesses of the human mind.

Jeffrey Dahmer

In the shadowed narratives of 20th-century serial killers, Jeffrey Dahmer's chilling tale stands out, not just for the horrific nature of his crimes but for the profound darkness that seemed to inhabit his very being. Dahmer, often referred to as the Milwaukee Cannibal, shocked the world with his admission to the murder and dismemberment of 17 young men and boys between 1978 and 1991. His gruesome acts didn't only involve killing; they incorporated deeply disturbing behaviors like necrophilia and cannibalism, repairing the façade of normality as he committed atrocities within the confines of his apartment.

Born on May 21, 1960, in Milwaukee, Wisconsin, Dahmer's early life appeared unremarkable, yet it hinted at the psychological complexities that would later manifest. His childhood was marred by a lack of attention from his parents, who were embroiled in their own tumultuous relationship. Some psychologists theorize that his increasing isolation and feelings of abandonment played a pivotal role in shaping his distorted psyche. Moreover, Dahmer's early fascination with animals, particularly their decomposition, seemed innocent until viewed in the chilling context of his future crimes.

As he entered adulthood, Dahmer's path became increasingly erratic and dangerous. He struggled with issues of sexuality and a compulsion for dominance and control. These underlying conflicts were exacerbated by alcohol dependence, which frequently left him disoriented and further isolated. Dahmer's killings were marked by an unsettling ritualistic aspect, capturing his victims with promises of money or companionship before drugging and eventually murdering them. His attempts to keep a part of them alive, whether through photographs or preserved body parts, underscore a deep-seated fear of abandonment and desire for control.

Arrested on July 22, 1991, Dahmer's reign of terror finally came to an end, largely due to the tenacity of one survivor. His trial, which captivated global media, offered a grim insight into the workings of the criminal mind. As experts debated Dahmer's sanity, the public grappled with a mix of revulsion and fascination. Convicted and sentenced to 15 life terms, Dahmer's life behind bars was cut short in 1994 when he was murdered by a fellow inmate, sealing his fate within the annals of infamy.

Analyzing Dahmer's life raises significant questions about the interplay between individual pathology and societal neglect. Was

Dahmer simply a product of his own mental aberrations, or did external factors play a pivotal role in his descent into darkness? While his story remains a terrifying chapter in the history of crime, it also serves as a stark reminder of the importance of understanding and addressing mental health issues before they escalate into avoidable tragedies.

In exploring the psyche of Jeffrey Dahmer, one can't help but reflect on the broader implications of his actions. As we strive to understand figures like him, we are drawn into a complex web of psychological, social, and moral inquiries. Each thread we untangle not only brings us closer to comprehending one man's terrifying legacy but also encourages us to more keenly scrutinize the shadows within our own communities.

John Wayne Gacy

John Wayne Gacy, often referred to as the "Killer Clown," stands as a chilling figure in the annals of criminal history. His facade was one of harmless joviality; he entertained children at parties, donning a clown costume and makeup. Yet, beneath this veneer lurked a predatory menace responsible for the gruesome murders of at least 33 young men and boys in the 1970s. Gacy's duality—his ability to mask savagery with charm—serves as a stark reminder of the complexity of the criminal mind.

Born in 1942, Gacy's early life was anything but idyllic. Raised in Chicago, he endured a tumultuous childhood marked by abuse and a turbulent relationship with his father. Some experts argue that Gacy's formative years shaped the deviant behaviors he would later exhibit. What drove him to become one of America's most infamous serial killers? A tangled web of psychological and environmental factors likely played a part. Despite a seemingly ordinary exterior, Gacy harbored deep-seated anger and desires that defied societal norms.

What is particularly haunting about Gacy is not just the sheer number of his victims but the methodical nature of his crimes. Many of his victims were vulnerable, lured from bus stations and seemingly safe environments under the guise of a job offer or favor. Gacy's ability to coax these young men to his suburban Chicago home speaks to his manipulative nature and the trust he could extract from those around him. Once inside, there was no escape. His basement turned into a chamber of horrors, where he committed acts of unspeakable brutality before hiding their bodies in the crawl space beneath his house.

Investigation into Gacy's crimes was initially slow. The victims' disappearances, while troubling, didn't immediately suggest a pattern. It took a confluence of concerned families, fledgling investigative techniques, and sheer determination by law enforcement to uncover the atrocities committed by Gacy. The breaking point came with the vanishing of 15-year-old Robert Piest, whose search led police to Gacy's doorstep and subsequently to the dreadful discovery beneath it.

His arrest and trial captivated the nation. The question of insanity loomed heavily, with the defense arguing psychological disturbance influenced Gacy's actions. However, the jury was unconvinced, and in 1980, they sentenced him to death. It was here, in the recounting of horrors at trial, that the public began to comprehend the extent of his malevolence. Gacy remained on death row for 14 years before meeting his fate via lethal injection in 1994. During this period, Gacy showed little remorse, often blaming his victims or claiming a split personality was responsible for his heinous acts.

Analyzing Gacy's life and crimes offers critical insights into the psychological makeup of serial killers. His case underscores the importance of understanding both environmental influences and inherent psychological disturbances, which together shape such predatory behavior. Though Gacy has long since been executed, the shadow he cast lingers, urging society to delve deeper into the mysterious and often terrifying recesses of the human psyche. The lessons learned from his case continue to inform criminal psychology and investigative practices today.

The Zodiac Killer

The Zodiac Killer left a haunting legacy that endures to this day, not least because the identity of the murderer remains a mystery. Active primarily in Northern California during the late 1960s and early 1970s, the Zodiac Killer claimed at least five confirmed victims, though he alleged to have murdered up to 37 people. What sets the Zodiac apart from other serial killers of his era is not just the brutality of the crimes, but his taunting communications with law enforcement and the media. Through cryptic letters and enigmatic ciphers sent to local newspapers, the killer turned the act of murder into a chilling game of cat-and-mouse.

The Zodiac's first confirmed attack occurred on December 20, 1968, when high school students Betty Lou Jensen and David Faraday were shot and killed near Vallejo, California. Just months later, on July 4, 1969, Darlene Ferrin and Michael Mageau were similarly attacked in a parking lot in Vallejo, though Mageau survived. These initial murders set the stage for a series of brazen acts that would confound law enforcement for years to come. The killer's boldness was exemplified by his phone calls to police, claiming responsibility for the attacks and providing details only the perpetrator would know.

The Zodiac's most alarming tactic was undoubtedly his meticulous ciphers, of which he sent four in total. These ciphers, filled with symbols and codes, were as much a riddle for the public as they were a dire warning. One of these was cracked in a week by a local schoolteacher and his wife, revealing a chilling message about the joy the killer found in murder. The most infamous of his puzzles, known as the 340 Cipher, went unsolved for over half a century before a team of amateur codebreakers deciphered it in 2020. This cipher, while not offering clues to his identity, did shed light on the callous nature of his psyche, revealing his desire to continue killing and his disdain for law enforcement efforts.

The Zodiac Killer's impact on popular culture cannot be overstated. He inspired numerous books, movies, and documentaries that have attempted to piece together the fragmented clues left in his wake. Authors and filmmakers often depict him as the epitome of evil masked in anonymity, a shadow that lurks just out of reach. His communications reveal a personality both cunning and conceited, one who reveled in the attention his actions garnered, yet one who deftly vanished whenever the net seemed to tighten.

In examining the mind of the Zodiac, several hypotheses have emerged over the years. Some experts believe he was a highly intelligent individual with a penchant for the spotlight. Others suggest a personality driven by deep-seated psychological issues, perhaps rooted in feelings of inadequacy or rejection. Despite numerous suspects over the years, none have been conclusively proven to be the Zodiac. This elusive phantom, who taunted authorities and terrified a nation, remains an enigma in the annals of criminal history, captivating the minds of armchair detectives and seasoned investigators alike. As the truth continues to hover achingly just beyond reach, the Zodiac Killer's specter reminds us of the dark complexities entrenched within the human psyche.

Richard Ramirez

Richard Ramirez, often referred to as the "Night Stalker," represents one of the most chilling figures in the annals of American crime. Born on February 29, 1960, in El Paso, Texas, Ramirez's life was a testament to the macabre, his sinister deeds casting a long shadow on the psyche of a city already fraught with fear. While his crimes spanned a mere year between 1984 and 1985, the brutality and randomness of his attacks have etched him into the grim roster of infamy among serial killers of the 20th century.

Ramirez's early life was a cauldron of violence, abuse, and dark influence. His older cousin, a Vietnam War veteran, boasted about his wartime atrocities and exposed young Richard to polaroids flaunting acts of extreme violence. This exposure seemed to unlock a primal urge in Ramirez, steering him toward a path of destruction. As is often noted in the study of serial killers, his childhood experiences were tumultuous, marked by physical abuse and inadequate boundaries, which contributed to his psychological unraveling.

By 1984, Los Angeles became his hunting ground. The crimes attributed to Ramirez were terrifyingly erratic; his victims were chosen without discernible pattern, spreading panic through communities. The breadth of his assaults ranged from burglary to rape to murder, and his methods were variably brutal, incorporating stabbing, beating, and shooting. Ramirez's lack of a consistent modus operandi made it challenging for law enforcement to connect the dots initially, leaving a trail of fear and confusion in his wake.

A chilling aspect of Ramirez was his satanic inclinations. He frequently left symbols of satanic worship at crime scenes and coerced his victims into professing their allegiance to Satan. This facet of his personality not only contributed to his notoriety but also illustrated a profound disconnect from societal norms and an embrace of chaos. This willingness to embody evil itself, aligning with the darkest aspects of human belief, lent a supernatural terror to his already horrific crimes.

In 1985, following a series of investigative breakthroughs, Ramirez was finally captured. A critical moment came when a fingerprint left at a stolen car linked him to a string of murders, ultimately leading to his arrest. The process was not without drama; Ramirez was apprehended by a mob of local residents after his identity was unveiled by the media, effectively marking the end of his reign of terror. His trial was a spectacle, revealing not just the extent of his crimes but the psychological chaos that propelled them.

The conviction of Ramirez resulted in 19 death sentences, a numerical testament to the magnitude of his depravity. His time on death row at San Quentin State Prison was marked by a mixture of defiance and celebrity, as he attracted a bizarre following of supporters, further testament to public fascination with the macabre. In 2013, his death from cancer closed the book on a life that had inflicted immeasurable suffering, but left behind questions that continue to haunt criminologists and psychologists alike.

Ultimately, Richard Ramirez's legacy is as much about the terror he instilled as it is about the broader societal fears he exposed. He left a nation grappling with the understanding that evil can sometimes walk among us unnoticed, acting as a cautionary tale about the fragile safety of the world we inhabit.

Albert DeSalvo

Albert DeSalvo's name became etched in the annals of American crime history largely due to the chilling moniker given to him: The Boston Strangler. His trail of terror in the early 1960s left an indelible mark on a city already grappling with the complexities of post-war society. Navigating the dingy streets of Boston, DeSalvo left behind a pattern of murders that were horrifying not just in act, but in their seeming randomness and brutality. He confessed to the strangling of 13 women, instilling a profound sense of fear and uncertainty among residents.

DeSalvo came from a troubled background, a facet common among notorious criminals of his ilk. Born in 1931, his childhood was marred by abuse and neglect. This tumultuous upbringing seemed to sow the seeds for his later violent behavior. His criminal activities began early in life, often centered around petty theft and burglary. Yet, as with many serial offenders, these initial transgressions proved to be a precursor to far graver crimes. The shift from mere theft to full-blown murder marked a dark evolution in his criminal career.

The public and authorities alike were perplexed by the psyche of DeSalvo. In a bid to understand the man behind the crimes, psychological profiles were drawn up, although they often skirted the deeper issues of mental illness and the lingering effects of his past. While DeSalvo was eventually apprehended for other offenses, it wasn't until he confessed to being the Boston Strangler that the full scope of his heinous acts came to light. Sentenced to life in prison, his admission was marred with controversy, as doubts lingered over the veracity of his confession and its implications.

Despite his confession, the debate over DeSalvo's guilt continues to this day, fueled by modern advancements in forensic science which in some cases dispute his involvement in several of the murders. Such uncertainty invites speculation: Was DeSalvo solely responsible, or were other perpetrators involved? This lingering question adds a layer of complexity to his story and challenges the competence of law enforcement tactics prevalent at the time.

In examining DeSalvo's reign of terror, one cannot overlook the role of the media in shaping the narrative. The sensationalistic portrayal of the Boston Strangler stoked public fear and drove an insatiable curiosity about the man behind the crimes. Within this whirlwind of conjecture and reportage, the true nature of Albert DeSalvo remains elusive, a specter in the shadowy intersection of reality and myth.

Albert DeSalvo's life and crimes offer a stark reflection on the sociocultural landscape of the time. His actions were a mirror to society's failings—questioning the effectiveness of the justice system, the influence of a tumultuous youth, and the dark potential lurking within a shattered psyche. It's a legacy that continues to puzzle psychologists, criminologists, and true crime enthusiasts, rendering the Boston Strangler an enigmatic figure in the macabre tapestry of 20th-century infamy.

Ed Gein

In the pantheon of American killers, Ed Gein holds a particularly grim distinction. Born in 1906 in rural Wisconsin, his life was marred by a deeply dysfunctional family dynamic, with his mother wielding a tyrannical influence over his worldview. Augusta Gein, a fervent Lutheran, instilled in Ed a fear and loathing of women, deeming them instruments of sin. This oppressive environment laid the groundwork for a psyche twisted by isolation and religious fanaticism.

Gein's criminal activities came to light in 1957 when local authorities were investigating the disappearance of Bernice Worden, a hardware store owner in Plainfield, Wisconsin. Their investigation led them to Gein's ramshackle farmhouse, a place shrouded in decay and palpable dread. What investigators found inside defied comprehension. Recovered were human artifacts created from corpses Gein had exhumed, alongside horrendous remnants of his victims. These grisly discoveries unearthed a macabre obsession with the female form, fixations stemming possibly from his intense hatred for yet desperate longing for his deceased mother.

Unlike more prolific killers, Gein's confirmed victim count stood at two: Mary Hogan and Bernice Worden. Yet, the horror of his crimes lay in the bizarre, theatrical nature of his actions, blurring the line between myth and reality in the annals of true crime. His morbid fascinations and the grotesque memorabilia found in his home would inspire fictional antagonists like Norman Bates of **Psycho** and Buffalo Bill of **The Silence of the Lambs**. These fictional iterations preserved

Gein's legacy, embedding him further into the cultural fabric as a symbol of unimaginable horror.

Psychologically, Gein was a conundrum—a man whose actions were motivated less by a desire to kill and more by a twisted attempt to resurrect the world he had lost with his mother's death. This facet of his psyche perplexed legal authorities and mental health professionals alike. Was Gein a cold-blooded killer or simply a man unable to grasp the horror of his actions, driven by a deranged perception of reality? His time in institutions for the criminally insane left this question largely unresolved, highlighting the complex interplay between mental illness and criminal culpability, a theme that resonates profoundly in the broader narrative of serial crime.

The legacy of Ed Gein extends beyond the atrocities he committed—he represents a psychological study that challenges our classic understanding of evil. His story compels us to ponder deeper questions about the influence of environment and upbringing in the formation of a killer's mindset. Is a man like Gein the product of nurture gone wrong, eternally warped by a pathological devotion to the memory of a domineering mother? Or is there something inherently sinister, a darkness lying dormant until conditions allow it to flourish? Gein's narrative invites us into a chilling contemplation of these questions.

Charles Manson

Charles Manson stands as one of the most notorious figures of the 20th century, not for his own hands-on involvement in the murders that shocked a nation, but for his unparalleled ability to manipulate and control. Manson's story is a dark narrative that intertwines elements of cultism, counter-culture, and a chilling charisma that drew people into his orbit. He wasn't a killer in the traditional sense but orchestrated a series of brutal murders that would forever embed him into the annals of criminal history.

Born in 1934 to a teenage mother, Manson's early years were tumultuous. Shuttled between relatives and often neglected, his childhood experiences laid a foundation of instability and rebellion. Manson spent much of his youth in and out of reformatory schools and institutions, where he honed his skills in manipulation and control. By the time he reached adulthood, he was adept at finding the vulnerable and exploiting them—skills that would become crucial in his later years.

During the 1960s, as America was engulfed in cultural revolution, Manson found himself drawn to the burgeoning hippie movement in California. Establishing what he called the "Manson Family", he managed to attract a group of devoted followers who saw him as a messianic figure. His ability to command his followers' loyalty was astonishing. Manson preached a distorted version of the coming apocalyptic race war, which he referred to as "Helter Skelter," drawing inspiration from music lyrics, especially those of The Beatles.

The summer of 1969 would mark a turning point. Under Manson's instruction, members of his cult brutally murdered actress Sharon Tate and four others at her Los Angeles home. The following nights saw the murders of Leno and Rosemary LaBianca. While Manson didn't commit the murders himself, his role as the mastermind behind these heinous acts implicates him fully in the eyes of justice. His control over the individuals who carried out these murders is a subject of continued intrigue and horror.

In a courtroom spectacle that captivated the nation, Manson was eventually found guilty of first-degree murder and conspiracy to commit murder. The trial was punctuated by strange outbursts and bizarre antics from Manson and his followers, further cementing his image as a man detached from ordinary human bounds. His prosecution was a pivotal moment in the intersection of media, crime, and public perception, highlighting the broader societal anxieties of the time.

Manson's life and crimes offer a labyrinthine glimpse into the capabilities of manipulation and the darkness that can reside within a charismatic person. Scholars and enthusiasts alike continue to delve into his psyche, trying to unravel the reasons behind his malevolent influence. What made Manson an enigma was not just his leadership of the Family but the psychological prowess he wielded to turn ordinary individuals into instruments of his dark vision.

Charles Manson died in 2017, but the spectral influence of his actions lingers. His legacy is a chilling reminder of how the boundaries between charisma and cruelty can sometimes blur, leading to catastrophic consequences. Manson's story continues to provoke questions about responsibility, control, and the darkest facets of human psychology.

David Berkowitz

The 1970s weren't just a time of disco and bell-bottoms; they birthed fear in New York City through the actions of David Berkowitz, notoriously known as the "Son of Sam." Berkowitz's reign of terror spanned from 1976 to 1977, creating a tense atmosphere throughout the city. During this period, his modus operandi was chillingly straightforward: approach unsuspecting young couples in parked cars and open fire with a .44 caliber Bulldog revolver. This pattern not only instilled fear but also left communities in a state of paralyzing anticipation. Each crime scene was a grim reminder of the unpredictability and randomness of his attacks.

The son of Jewish adoptive parents, Berkowitz struggled with his identity and feelings of abandonment from a young age. This tumultuous start in life laid the groundwork for his later psychological breakdowns. Growing up in the Bronx, his early life seemed fairly ordinary on the surface. However, beneath this veneer, he battled demons that only he could see and hear. Berkowitz claimed his neighbor's dog was possessed by a demon commanding him to kill, leading to a bizarre yet terrifying narrative that became part of his identity in the public eye.

Psychologists and law enforcement professionals have since dissected his twisted psyche, trying to make sense of his motivations. Berkowitz exhibited many of the classic signs found in later serial killers: cruelty to animals, arson, and a troubled family life. Yet, what made him unique was his attention-grabbing communication style. The letters he left at his murder scenes were taunting, filled with a craving for attention and a desire to instill panic. These letters were not only addressed to the police but also the media, fuelling a media frenzy that plastered his alias across the headlines.

Investigations into Berkowitz's murders met initial challenges, largely due to the lack of advanced forensic technology at the time. The police, however, developed a task force specifically designed to catch him. It was a parking ticket, registered near the site of one of his attacks, that eventually led to his capture. In August 1977, Berkowitz was apprehended, bringing relief to a city held hostage by fear. During his trial, his declarations of demonic influence played a role in shaping public debate around insanity and accountability in the judicial process.

Even after his incarceration, Berkowitz remains a figure of fascination and horror. He has claimed a religious rebirth in prison and expressed remorse for his actions. Yet, the shadows of his deeds linger on, prevalent reminders within both criminal psychology studies and the broader narrative of American serial killers. The case of David Berkowitz underscores the complexity of dissecting criminal minds, merging elements of psychology, criminal justice, and media influence in a macabre dance that continues to captivate the world today.

In the grand tapestry of infamous killers, Berkowitz stands as a poignant example of the terror one individual can inflict on a sprawling metropolis. His story serves as both a warning and a puzzle—a dark reflection on the possibilities of human nature turned malevolent.

Dennis Rader

Dennis Rader, perhaps better known by his infamous moniker the BTK Killer, presents a chilling case study in the deceptive ordinariness often found in some of the 20th century's most notorious killers. Operating under the radar for decades, Rader managed to commit heinous crimes while simultaneously leading what appeared to be a normal suburban life in Wichita, Kansas. His story is a stark reminder of the duality that can exist within a criminal mind: the ability to mask monstrous intentions behind the veneer of everyday existence.

Born in 1945, Rader's trajectory into infamy wasn't immediately evident. He was an Air Force veteran, a family man, and even a Boy Scout leader. His public persona was that of a diligent worker and church council president. Yet, beneath this facade lay a malevolent nature driven by an insidious desire for control and domination. Rader coined his own title, BTK, which stood for "bind, torture, kill," a methodical manifesto of his approach to violence. Each aspect of this acronym reveals the cold, calculated nature of his crimes— meticulously planned and executed with a level of detachment that's as disturbing as it is incomprehensible.

Between 1974 and 1991, Rader's trail of terror included the murders of ten individuals. His victims, ranging from age 9 to 62, were selected without any discernible pattern beyond proximity and opportunity. This randomness contributed to the pervasive fear he instilled in the Wichita community. Despite his spree during these years, Rader managed to evade capture, a testament to both his cunning and the limitations of investigative technology at the time. It wasn't until 2005, long after his last known murder, that law enforcement finally apprehended him after he reignited communication with authorities—a move that ultimately led to his downfall.

Rader's capture was a catalyst for reflection on the evolution of criminal profiling and forensic science. Investigators utilized advancements in DNA technology, which had progressed significantly since his initial crimes. A pivotal moment came when DNA collected from Rader's daughter's medical records provided the match needed to link him to the crime scenes. His arrest and subsequent confession brought some closure to the families affected, yet also elicited broader societal questions about the nature of evil and its ability to hide in plain sight.

Perhaps most chilling is Rader's lack of remorse. During his trial, Rader recounted his crimes with a disturbing detachment, offering a glimpse into the psychological abyss characteristic of many serial killers. His candid admissions and seemingly emotionless demeanor force us to confront the uncomfortable truth that such individuals exist amongst us. They challenge our understanding of morality and the human psyche, leaving us to ponder whether true rehabilitation is possible for those devoid of empathy.

In the annals of criminal history, Dennis Rader stands as a perplexing figure—a killer who thrived on the notoriety he cultivated, yet whose public capture and confession laid bare the innate vulnerabilities in his need for validation. His story not only underscores the critical role of advancements in forensics and investigative technique improvements but also serves as a poignant reminder of the importance of vigilance and heightened awareness in the ongoing battle against such insidious threats.

Harold Shipman

Harold Shipman, a name etched into the annals of infamy, stands out among the most notorious killers of the 20th century. Known as "Dr. Death," Shipman didn't fit the typical serial killer profile; he was a respected general practitioner, a trusted figure in the community of Hyde, England. People welcomed him into their homes, seeking care and comfort from a man whose profession should have been the opposite of his clandestine vocation. In reality, Shipman's outward facade masked a chilling career of murder, positioning him as possibly the most prolific serial killer in modern history.

What sets Shipman apart from other infamous killers of his time was his methodical approach and choice of weapon—morphine. As a doctor, he had unfettered access to the drug and a trusted position that facilitated his horrors. From the late 1970s to 1998, Shipman is believed to have killed at least 250 of his patients, predominantly older women. He conveniently labeled many deaths as natural, exploiting his role to obliterate suspicion for years. His victims were often found sitting peacefully, a grim testament to the silent efficiency of his murderous methods.

The veneer began to crack in 1998 when the daughter of one of his victims, Kathleen Grundy, expressed doubts about her mother's will, which suspiciously named Shipman as the primary beneficiary. The anomaly brought Shipman's murderous pastime into the spotlight for the first time. A subsequent inquiry revealed evidence of tampered records and damning traces of morphine in exhumed bodies. He was convicted in 2000 of 15 murders, but this was just the tip of the iceberg.

Shipman's capture initiated a wider investigation that unearthed chilling patterns of his crimes, prompting a painstaking review of thousands of patient records. It became clear that Shipman's capabilities as a doctor had been morphed into a lethal advantage; he knew how to kill without drawing attention, and how to cover his tracks with clinical precision.

This case not only shook the medical community but also exposed glaring inadequacies in the oversight of professionals in positions of trust. The Shipman Inquiry, which followed his conviction, brought urgent reforms in medical regulations. In many ways, Harold Shipman was a wake-up call for systemic change. It served as a grim reminder of how the lines between healer and harmer could be devastatingly thin when oversight fails.

The reasons behind Shipman's actions remain largely speculative, an enigmatic puzzle of power, control, and perhaps a deep-seated compulsion that defies traditional understanding. His case continues to challenge criminologists and psychologists who attempt to decipher the darkness that overshadowed his professional oath. Ultimately, Harold Shipman represents a haunting dichotomy—how a man's sworn duty to save lives was perverted into a furtive spree of unparalleled death.

Aileen Wuornos

Aileen Wuornos remains one of the most infamous female serial killers of the 20th century. Her life was a tapestry woven from threads of abuse, abandonment, and chaos, and it culminated in a series of murders that would shock the world. Wuornos's trajectory into the dark annals of criminal history was influenced by a host of environmental and psychological factors that transformed her life into a potent case study for both law enforcement and psychologists.

Born in Rochester, Michigan, Wuornos's childhood was marred with instability. Abandoned by her mother and later experiencing profound neglect, she never had a stable home base. She turned to the streets at an early age, trading her body for basic necessities and grasping at anything to survive. This formative experience shaped her perception of relationships and placed her on a path that mingled desperation with violence.

Her tumultuous romantic relationships reflected a deeper psychological unease, a search for affection that always seemed maddeningly out of reach. Wuornos's crimes can't be separated from her fractured psyche. Her killings, committed between 1989 and 1990, targeted men who solicited her services as a sex worker. She claimed self-defense, asserting that she killed these men to protect herself from sexual assault. While the authenticity of this defense is debated, it underscores the complex interplay of vulnerability and violence in her life.

The media painted Wuornos as a "man-hating" predator, amplifying the sensational aspects of her gender and methodology. Society's morbid fascination with her case lay partly in her deviation from the typical profiles of male serial killers. Female serial killers are relatively rare, and Wuornos's visibility forced a reevaluation of gender dynamics within serial crime.

Wuornos's trial and subsequent execution in 2002 highlighted key tensions within the judicial system, particularly in cases involving mental illness and the death penalty. Her erratic behavior and explosive courtroom outbursts demonstrated a fractured mind, sparking debates about her mental fitness and accountability. These discussions remain critical as they echo broader dialogues about the role of mental illness in criminal behavior and the ethics of capital punishment for those deemed mentally unstable.

Despite the chilling nature of her crimes, Wuornos's life and choices prompt vital questions about the intersection of nature and nurture. Her story suggests that her actions were not just the result of innate malevolence but were influenced by her deeply troubled past. It's a tale that prompts introspection on our societal responsibilities to those who, pushed to the margins, may develop into something unfathomable.

Ultimately, Aileen Wuornos's life and crimes serve as a stark reminder of how personal demons, left unchecked, can manifest into horrendous acts. Her story is a confluence of tragedy and menace, raising crucial questions about prevention, intervention, and justice. In exploring Wuornos's life, one grapples not only with the atrocities she committed but also with the existential underpinnings that society must reckon with to prevent future horrors. In understanding Wuornos, perhaps we can glean insights into the fractured paths of others who might otherwise follow in her footsteps.

Andrei Chikatilo

In the shadowy world of serial killers, few names inspire the same level of dread as Andrei Chikatilo. Known as the "Butcher of Rostov," Chikatilo's heinous crimes in Soviet Russia during the last decades of the 20th century are chilling reminders of the depths of human depravity. Born in Ukraine in 1936, Chikatilo's early life was marked by profound hardships, including famine and political upheaval, circumstances that arguably sowed the seeds of his later monstrosity. However, it wasn't until much later in life that Chikatilo's dark proclivities began to manifest in unimaginable acts of violence.

Chikatilo's reign of terror began in the late 1970s, stretching over a dozen years, during which he brutally murdered more than 50 women and children. Utilizing a persona of unassuming normalcy, he lured his victims with promises of food, shelter, or employment, often preying upon society's most vulnerable. His killings, marked by extreme violence and sexual assault, left communities in a state of terror and bewilderment, particularly due to the lack of clear motive beyond an insatiable appetite for cruelty.

The Soviet Union of the 1980s was rife with bureaucratic inefficiencies, and Chikatilo took full advantage of this chaos. Law enforcement's handling of his case was plagued by missteps and delays, partially compounded by a system that was reluctant to acknowledge the possibility of a serial killer in its midst. This climate allowed Chikatilo to evade capture for years, yet his actions also catalyzed one of the most extensive manhunts in Soviet history. Investigators were tasked with an enormous challenge, piecing together fragments of evidence in an era before advanced forensic tools were readily available.

The psychological aspects of Chikatilo's crimes present a compelling case study. Described by clinical psychologists as incapable of controlling his violent impulses, Chikatilo claimed his physical impairments and childhood traumas drove his notorious actions. Some experts suggest his inability to perform sexually contributed to his overwhelming need to dominate and destroy. While these factors offer insight, they hardly justify the scale of violence he inflicted. Instead, they underscore the complexities of dissecting a criminal psyche intertwined with deep-seated mental illness.

Chikatilo's capture in 1990 marked a turning point. A combination of persistent police work and emerging behavioral profiling techniques finally led to his arrest. Upon interrogation, his confessions shed light on the intricate details of his crimes, which were as methodical as they were savage. During his highly publicized trial, Chikatilo exhibited erratic behavior, leading to questions about his sanity. Nonetheless, he was found guilty and executed in 1994, closing a chapter of one of the Soviet Union's most harrowing criminal episodes.

Ultimately, Chikatilo's legacy is a haunting reminder of the darkness that can lurk beneath a seemingly ordinary facade. The efforts to apprehend him brought about significant advancements in forensic science and criminal profiling in Russia. As criminologists and historians continue to analyze his life and crimes, the story of Andrei Chikatilo remains a crucial lesson in both the dangers of overlooking early warning signs and the relentless pursuit of justice in the face of unspeakable evil.

Pedro LÃ³pez

The desolate terrains of Colombia, Peru, and Ecuador became the playground for one of the most prolific and enigmatic serial killers of the 20th century—Pedro Alonso López. Dubbed the "Monster of the Andes," López operated in the shadows, his horrific deeds known only to a few until his arrests and subsequent confessions shone a grim light on his unsettling psyche. His story isn't merely one of heinous crimes; it represents a chilling intersection of personal trauma and societal negligence.

López's early life was marred by severe trauma and neglect. Born in 1948 in Colombia, his childhood was a nightmare of abuse and homelessness. His mother's alleged neglect and his exposure to street violence provided the initial fuel for the rage simmering within him. At a young age, López was reportedly expelled from home, only to find himself in the brutal environs of the street. This early exposure to violence and survival at any cost forged a personality that would eventually see human life as trivial.

By adulthood, López's path had distorted into a grotesque trajectory of violence. His vultures of choice were young girls, numbering into the hundreds, as he confessed. Tragically, many of their bodies remain undiscovered, scattered across the desolate landscapes where he operated with impunity. The authorities' initial reluctance to acknowledge the scope of his crimes played directly into his hands, enabling him to continue his spree for far longer than should have been possible. His modus operandi remained consistent—isolating vulnerable children, often from indigenous communities, capitalizing on their invisibility to execute his plans without repercussion.

The narrative takes an even more disturbing turn upon López's arrest. In 1980, his capture in Ecuador uncovered the horrific extent of his crimes. However, his conviction and sentencing to just 16 years in prison—due to Ecuador's then-lax laws on murder—brought international outrage. His early release in 1994 after only 14 years, for "good behavior," stands as a stark testament to the inadequacies of the justice system dealing with crimes of this magnitude. Not long after, López vanished, practically disappearing from official view and leaving questions about his potential ongoing threat unanswered.

Despite his monstrous acts, understanding López also requires a look at the socio-political environment that failed both him as a child and his victims. The socio-economic disparities in the regions he targeted created an ideal environment for his brand of terror. López essentially exploited a system that neglected its most vulnerable, pointing to a broader systemic issue that extends beyond one killer's gruesome undertakings.

The Pedro López case continues to haunt criminologists and psychologists today. It serves as a potent illustration of what happens when personal trauma, social neglect, and law enforcement shortcomings collide. Analyzing his actions forces introspection on the effectiveness of justice and social welfare systems, as well as the chilling reality that, even today, there might still be 'monsters' lurking somewhere, either caught in the making or waiting to be unleashed by the same set of failures.

Gary Ridgway

Gary Ridgway, infamously known as the "Green River Killer," stands as a chilling figure in the annals of American crime. Operating in the Seattle area, Ridgway's reign of terror began in the early 1980s and lasted for almost two decades. His nickname derives from the Green River, where the bodies of his first known victims were discovered. The level of his brutality and the sheer number of victims place him among the most prolific serial killers in U.S. history. Ridgway's ability to evade capture for so long was facilitated by his outwardly unremarkable facade; a seemingly normal man who blended seamlessly into his surroundings. His case presents a haunting study of contradiction: an outward appearance of normalcy that hid a monstrous proclivity for violence.

The enormity of Ridgway's crimes was staggering. By his own admission, he claimed responsibility for the murders of over 70 women, though he's been convicted for 49. Ridgway's victims were often vulnerable women, many of whom were sex workers. This choice served a chilling practicality: marginalized by society, many of his victims lacked a support network that would mobilize quickly when they disappeared. To Ridgway, these women were not only easy targets but also human voids that he could exploit, and then dispose of, with little fear of immediate retribution.

Ridgway's psychological profile paints a picture of a remorseless predator. He exhibited traits common among many serial killers—manipulation, deceit, and a lack of empathy. Yet, what makes Ridgway particularly disturbing is his calculated patience. Unlike many of his counterparts who thrived on chaos and impulsivity, Ridgway operated with chilling methodical precision. He often strangled his victims, a method that required close contact and significant time, suggesting a need for dominance and control. Furthermore, Ridgway would return to the scenes to have intercourse with the bodies of his victims, revealing a complex and deeply disturbed psyche that thrived on revisiting the locus of his power.

Despite numerous interviews and confessions, much of Ridgway's inner world remains elusive. What drove him to such heinous acts? Though various psychologists have speculated about deep-seated issues, such as abnormal family dynamics and sexual dysfunction, Ridgway's rationalizations were often disturbing in their simplicity. He articulated his actions as a consequence of convenience rather than compulsion, claiming he considered murder akin to a utility to eliminate prostitutes whom he felt were unnecessary in society.

The investigation into Ridgway's killing spree stretched across two decades, stymied by a lack of forensic evidence and the transient lifestyles of his victims. It wasn't until the advent of DNA profiling that authorities were finally able to link Ridgway to the murders decisively. His arrest in 2001 marked the end of one of America's most prolonged manhunts, shining a spotlight on the advancements in forensic science but also on the failures that allowed him to go undetected for so long.

Gary Ridgway's case continues to serve as a grim reminder of the human capacity for darkness and the complex tapestry of societal, psychological, and procedural factors that allow such heinous crimes to occur. It prompts an ongoing conversation about the vulnerabilities of marginalized communities, the evolving landscape of criminal investigation, and the ceaseless endeavor to understand—and ultimately prevent—the emergence of such relentless predators.

Edmund Kemper

Edmund Kemper, a towering figure both literally and figuratively in the annals of criminal history, invites profound inquiry for those curious about the darkest edges of psychological deviance. Standing at 6 feet 9 inches, Kemper is not only notable for his physical stature but also for the gruesome acts that earned him infamy. His story weaves a complex narrative of formative experiences, opportunistic violence, and chilling introspection.

Born in California in 1948, Kemper's tumultuous childhood laid a foundation for his later violent outbursts. His troubled relationship with his mother, Clarnell Strandberg, constantly simmered in a concoction of abuse and manipulation. Clarnell's relentless belittling and emotional torment sowed seeds of deep resentment in young Kemper. As he grew, these feelings gestated into a profound animosity towards women, a recurring theme that emerged during his later crimes.

Kemper's criminal career began early. At the age of 15, he murdered his grandparents, an act he described as a means to experience what killing felt like. Institutionalized in a state hospital, he was subsequently released at 21, deemed rehabilitated by the very institutions meant to safeguard society. Underneath the veneer of improved behavior, however, Kemper's darker impulses lay in wait.

Between 1972 and 1973, Kemper embarked on a killing spree that targeted young women—hitchhikers who fell victim to his perverse fantasies. His modus operandi involved not just murder but acts of necrophilia and dismemberment. Kemper's intelligence and manipulative prowess allowed him to evade capture for an unsettlingly long time, underscoring a chilling proficiency in exploiting human trust.

Perhaps what separates Kemper from other serial killers is his candidness post-apprehension. After murdering his mother and her friend in April 1973, he turned himself in to the authorities. Kemper's willingness to collaborate with investigators provided rare insights into the psyche of a serial killer, revealing a level of self-awareness that is both shocking and invaluable to criminal psychologists.

Analyzing Kemper's confessions, experts identified notable psychopathic traits aligned with subsequent manipulative behaviors. Despite the horrific nature of his crimes, he demonstrated a peculiar logic behind his actions, offering a rare glimpse into the mind of a calculated predator. Kemper's interviews with psychiatrist and author Margaret Cheney further fed public fascination, as his articulate reflections seemed inexplicably at odds with the brutality of his acts.

The legacy of Edmund Kemper is multifaceted, resonating in the fields of criminal psychology and law enforcement. His case prompted discussions about early intervention and the rehabilitation of youthful offenders. Kemper's life and crimes serve as a stark reminder of the potential consequences when psychological red flags are ignored. As his story continues to capture the imaginations of true crime enthusiasts, Kemper remains a chilling testament to the violent intersections of nature, nurture, and opportunity.

Peter Sutcliffe

Peter Sutcliffe, infamously known as the Yorkshire Ripper, stands among the ranks of 20th-century killers who etched fear into the public consciousness. His reign of terror in the late 1970s and early 1980s left a trail of suffering and death across northern England, where his modus operandi targeted vulnerable women, igniting a societal frenzy that rippled far beyond the crime scenes.

Sutcliffe's early life did not outwardly signal his eventual descent into violence. Born in 1946 in Bingley, West Yorkshire, he came from a working-class family with nominal interest in academics but a penchant for solitude. Early employment as a gravedigger and truck driver served as a veneer of normality, but it was during these formative years that psychological fissures began to show.

His violent spree commenced in 1975, a time when Sutcliffe's misogynistic rage took shape, driven by a delusional belief that he was on a mission ordained by divine forces. In the ensuing years, his attacks became more brutal and methodical. Concealing his identity under the cover of night, Sutcliffe inflicted horror on unsuspecting victims, primarily targeting sex workers, a choice that reflected deep-seated prejudices and contributed to the challenges faced by investigators.

The investigation into the Yorkshire Ripper case marked a pivotal moment in British criminology. As the body count rose, so did public pressure and criticism of law enforcement's handling of the case. A myriad of factors, from procedural errors to the infamous "Wearside Jack" hoax, hampered the pursuit of justice. Despite extensive evidence and multiple interviews, Sutcliffe's capture remained elusive for several years, highlighting the imperfect art of criminal profiling at the time.

The eventual breakthrough came in January 1981, when Sutcliffe's misstep—a vehicle registration irregularity—led to his arrest. During subsequent interrogations, he confessed to the murders, revealing details that were as chilling as they were appalling. Sutcliffe's mental state was a focal point during his trial, where his defense hinged on claims of paranoid schizophrenia. However, the court convicted him of murder, sentencing him to life imprisonment—a decision reflecting the gravity of his crimes despite his mental health arguments.

Sutcliffe's legacy extends beyond his own narrative, serving as a cautionary tale of systemic failures and the complexities of the criminal mind. The Yorkshire Ripper case instigated significant changes within the British police force, triggering reforms in investigative techniques and approaches to victimology, which continue to influence modern policing.

Over time, Peter Sutcliffe's story has been dissected through numerous mediums, from documentaries to academic inquiries, each seeking to understand what tethered together the strands of his fractured psyche. In examining Sutcliffe's haunting impact, one uncovers the eternal struggle to reconcile human cruelty with the pursuit of justice—a theme that resonates across the chronicles of history's most infamous criminals.

Ian Brady and Myra Hindley

In the annals of 20th-century crime, the names Ian Brady and Myra Hindley evoke an unsettling sense of dread. Known as the Moors Murderers, their partnership in crime made them one of the most notorious killer duos in history. Between July 1963 and October 1965, they abducted, tortured, and murdered five children, burying their small bodies in the bleak expanses of Saddleworth Moor in northwest England. The sheer depravity of their acts shocked a nation and left an indelible mark on Britain's collective psyche.

Brady and Hindley's macabre alliance began in 1961 when they met while working at a chemical company in Manchester. Brady, possessing a chillingly cold demeanor, was a self-described nihilist. He drew Hindley into a world of gruesome fantasies, influenced by his obsession with Nazi Germany and the writings of the Marquis de Sade. Hindley, enamored with Brady and desperate for his approval, became a willing accomplice. This sinister bond formed the bedrock of their crimes, with Hindley often luring the victims into Brady's trap.

Their first victim, Pauline Reade, was just 16 when she vanished, setting off an unfolding horror. The murders followed a chilling pattern: abduction, abuse, and murder, with the scenes recorded in photographs and audio recordings. The trial of Brady and Hindley, in 1966, unveiled a gruesome narrative to the public, with Hindley's mugshot becoming an unsettling icon of evil. The evidence, particularly audio recordings of victim Lesley Ann Downey's final moments, left the jury and the public in shock.

The psychological dynamics between Brady and Hindley continue to intrigue criminologists and psychologists. Was Hindley a victim of manipulation, or did she harbor her own dark motives? Their relationship, a toxic blend of domination and complicity, raises questions about the nature of influence and shared criminal intent. Such partnerships challenge conventional understandings of individual culpability, blurring lines between puppet and puppeteer in the theatre of crime.

Their capture resulted from a break in their carefully constructed façade. David Smith, Hindley's brother-in-law, witnessed the aftermath of their final murder and alerted the police, leading to the duo's arrest. Despite being convicted of three murders initially, Brady and Hindley's true body count and the extent of their crimes remained subjects of speculation for decades. Brady's psychological manipulations did not end with his incarceration; he spent much of his life attempting to exert control and gain infamy even from behind bars.

Brady and Hindley's case holds vital lessons for criminal psychology and investigative strategies. Their crimes demonstrated how closely entwined motivations and methods could be when two disturbed minds align. The case forced British law enforcement and the public to grapple with the human capacity for evil and the dangers of idolizing figures, even among criminal skies. It serves as a grim reminder of the importance of vigilance and the potentially catastrophic consequences when warning signs are ignored.

The legacy of Ian Brady and Myra Hindley is a dark chapter in criminal history that poses uncomfortable questions about the depths of human depravity. Yet, by examining these infamous killers, we gain insight not just into their twisted psyches but also into the mechanisms of justice and the importance of preventing such atrocities from unfolding again.

Fred and Rosemary West

In the grim annals of British crime, Fred and Rosemary West stand as chilling figures of depravity and cruelty. Their story, initially hidden by the veneer of a seemingly normal life, gradually unfolded into a nightmare that rivaled the haunting tales of any horror story. The Wests' home at 25 Cromwell Street in Gloucester, later dubbed the "House of Horrors," became the final resting place for many of their victims, the site of unspeakable acts that bespoke the depths of human depravity.

Fred West was born into a turbulent environment, one where violence and abuse were constant spectres. Psychological assessments suggest his early experiences blinded him to moral boundaries, laying a foundation for a life marked by brutality. Fred's marriage to Rosemary Letts in 1972 formed a partnership not just in life but in crime. Rosemary, sharing an equally troubled upbringing marked by neglect and abuse, emerged as a willing participant in Fred's grim ventures. What they did together over the years defies the very essence of humanity.

The Wests' modus operandi often involved luring young women to their home with promises of work or a place to stay. Once inside, these victims faced unimaginable horrors. They were subjected to prolonged captivity, sexual abuse, and eventually, murder. Fred meticulously buried some of the victims in the cellar, while others were interred in the garden. Each discovery during the police investigation revealed the depth of their heinous acts, painting a ghastly picture of life and death within their walls.

It's crucial to understand how Fred and Rosemary complemented each other's sadistic tendencies. Fred, often depicted as the more dominant figure, would conduct much of the physical torment. Rosemary, far from a passive accomplice, engaged actively in the abuse, her cruelty as profound and chilling as Fred's. Their synergy turned them into one of the most notorious killer duos of the 20th century. It

43

raises harrowing questions about the nature of evil and partnership in crime; when two destructive forces collaborate, the results can be catastrophically amplified.

The unraveling of their crimes began in 1992 after the police investigated the disappearance of their daughter, Heather. Her disappearance, alongside mounting allegations of abuse from other family members, led to a full-scale investigation. What the authorities uncovered, hidden within the depths of 25 Cromwell Street, shocked the nation. The unearthing of human remains kickstarted a complex legal battle, ultimately leading to Fred's suicide while awaiting trial and Rosemary's life imprisonment.

The case of Fred and Rosemary West is more than just a chronicle of barbarity. It serves as a study in pathology, offering insights into how certain environments and relationships can nurture the worst in human behavior. Discussions around their psychological profiles contribute to the broader understanding of criminal minds, challenging experts to reconcile the monstrous acts with the complex interplay of nurture, nature, and personal choice. Their legacy is a grim reminder of the darkness that can lurk beneath the surface of normality, and the importance of vigilance in recognizing the signs before it's too late.

John Allen Muhammad and Lee Boyd Malvo

In the autumn chill of 2002, fear cloaked the Washington D.C. metropolitan area as a series of seemingly random sniper shootings began to unravel. This grim chapter was none other than the terror orchestrated by John Allen Muhammad and his young accomplice, Lee Boyd Malvo. They embarked on a killing spree that left ten people dead and several others wounded over a span of three weeks. Their motives, shrouded in a mix of personal vendettas and a distorted sense of righteousness, perplexed investigators and fueled public panic.

Muhammad, a Gulf War veteran, brought a sense of military precision to their attacks. He adopted a ruthless methodology, evoking a chilling atmosphere of unpredictability. His influence over Malvo, a teenager at the time, was significant. They shared a twisted father-son dynamic, with Malvo viewing Muhammad as a mentor and a father figure, despite the much darker undertones of their relationship. This dynamic amplified the psychological complexity of the duo, blurring the lines between coercion and collaboration.

The duo transformed an innocuous blue Chevrolet Caprice into a mobile sniper's nest, fashioning a hole in the trunk to conceal their deadly intentions. This sinister innovation allowed them to carry out their attacks with stealth, striking from a seemingly invisible vantage point. The public, caught in the web of fear, was incapacitated by a growing dread of everyday activities, from pumping gas to walking across parking lots. Their ability to meld into the urban landscape and become virtually undetectable made the pursuit one of increasing urgency for law enforcement.

The psychology behind their murderous spree is as enigmatic as the crimes themselves. For Muhammad, the incentives seemed to stew in a cauldron of personal grievances, ideological extremism, and a thirst for manipulation. Malvo, on the other hand, was drawn into this lethal partnership through a combination of manipulation and admiration. Cognitive pathways distorted by Muhammad's guidance led Malvo down a dark road, where each act of violence was framed as part of a macabre apprenticeship.

The culmination of their reign of terror came to an end on October 24, 2002, when they were apprehended at a rest stop in Maryland. The pair were discovered sleeping in their car, the weapon of choice—a Bushmaster rifle—lying in the vehicle. Their capture was the result of a massive investigative effort that pieced together tiny fragments of evidence, including ballistics, eyewitness accounts, and vehicle sightings, culminating in a mosaic that finally revealed the killers' identities.

Once in custody, their trials unfolded to reveal the depths of their crimes and the complexities of their motivations. Muhammad received a death sentence and was executed by lethal injection in 2009. Malvo, considered by many to be a product of Muhammad's manipulation, was sentenced to life imprisonment without parole. His case ignites ongoing debates about the influence of age and indoctrination on criminal accountability.

The story of John Allen Muhammad and Lee Boyd Malvo is not just a tale of horror and loss, but a profound reflection on the human psyche's vulnerabilities to influence and radicalization. Their narrative threads into the broader tapestry of 20th-century crimes, where the lines between predator and prey, innocence and culpability, remain indelibly blurred.

Albert Fish

Albert Fish, a name that resonates with a chilling whisper in the annals of true crime history, stands out as one of the most grotesquely infamous killers of the 20th century. Born Hamilton Howard Fish in 1870, his life was marked by unspeakable acts of depravity blended with a veneer of normalcy that belied his true nature. Fish's story is one that traverses the boundaries of horror, delving into the depths of a disturbed mind that was somehow capable of functioning under societal norms.

Growing up, Fish was engulfed in a tumultuous environment—an element that would inevitably sculpt his future proclivities. His childhood was marred by abandonment and instability, his father dying young and his mother placing him in an orphanage where he was subject to severe strife and abuse. These early experiences likely laid the foundation for his later crimes, seeding the sadistic tendencies that would emerge in horrific fashion.

Fish's adult life played out as a disturbing continuation of the traumas he endured in youth. He developed an obsessive interest in pain and punishment, a macabre fascination that spiraled into his criminal exploits. His outward appearance, however, was that of an innocuous elderly gentleman, a disguise that enabled him to evade suspicion and enact his unspeakable deeds under a cloak of deceptive gentility.

The depravity of Fish's actions found its apex in the infamous case of Grace Budd. In 1928, Fish kidnapped and brutally murdered the young girl, an act which he would later detail with chilling precision in a letter to her family. This brutal crime, coupled with his bizarre and violent proclivities, led to his moniker as the 'Brooklyn Vampire'. It was the calculated normalcy in his communication that horrified the public and brought shocking clarity to his persona.

Fish's eventual capture shed light on an extensive history of heinous acts, including claims of cannibalism. His trial, fraught with sensationalism, captivated the nation. Experts delved into the depths of his psyche, calling him a "psychiatric phenomenon". Yet, many questions lingered about what truly drove his pathological behavior. Was it pure evil or a concoction of mental derangement, formed by his sordid past?

Despite the heinous nature of his crimes, Fish's case contributed significantly to the evolution of forensic psychiatry. It propelled discussions on the intersections of mental illness and criminality, challenging the judicial system to grapple with the balance between culpability and insanity. Examining Fish's sickening legacy provides stark insights into the evil capabilities of the human mind, as well as the societal factors that can cultivate such monstrosity.

In the broader narrative of infamy that characterizes 20th-century killers, Albert Fish presents one of the most unsettling chapters. His grim tale remains a testament to the complex interplay of psychology and crime, where the abyss of the human mind often holds more questions than answers, showcasing the perpetual challenge faced by those seeking to understand—and prevent—the emergence of such terrifying figures.

Richard Speck

In the annals of 20th-century crime, Richard Speck commands a chilling entry, not for the intricacies of his methods, but for the sheer brutality and randomness of his crimes. The sweltering night of July 13, 1966, became his macabre canvas. Speck invaded a South Chicago townhouse that served as a dormitory for nursing students and unleashed a savagery that would shake the nation. By morning, eight young women lay dead, the victims of an unfathomable rampage. Only one survived, hiding her terror until the dawn, ultimately to become the solitary witness to Speck's horror.

Richard Speck's life was marked by instability and violence long before this infamous night. Born in Kirkwood, Illinois, in 1941, Speck faced a turbulent childhood characterized by an abusive stepfather and constant family upheavals. These early influences cannot be understated when considering the formation of his violent tendencies. His adolescent years saw the beginning of a rap sheet filled with petty crimes, foreshadowing his later descent into more serious offenses. Suspended between anger and alienation, Speck wandered through his early adulthood, a ticking time bomb of resentment and frustration.

The night of the murders, Speck was reportedly under the influence of both alcohol and drugs, substances that blurred the lines between reality and nightmare. However, for all the haze, his actions were terrifyingly deliberate. He bound and attacked each victim, moving from room to room as if driven by an unstoppable force. The path he carved through that townhouse is not simply the story of a violent spree; it's a troubling snapshot of a man who had relinquished his humanity. Speck's method of operation—impulsive yet chillingly systematic—underscores the unpredictable nature of his personality. He did not fit neatly into established profiles of serial killers, his motives muddied by the fury boiling inside him.

Speck's capture and trial made headlines around the world, casting a shadow over the city of Chicago. Forensic experts and psychologists delved into what lay behind Speck's eyes, eyes that flickered between defiance and detachment throughout his court proceedings. The trial raised significant questions about the intersection of mental illness, substance abuse, and criminal accountability. Speck himself offered little clarity, alternating between expressions of remorse and bitter resignation, leaving jurors and the public to speculate on the true nature of his guilt.

Speck was sentenced to death, although his sentence was later commuted to life imprisonment following the abolition of the death penalty in Illinois. During his time in prison, he remained a figure of both fear and fascination, his life behind bars offering occasional glimpses into the mind of a man who had nothing left to lose. Notoriously, a 1996 video surfacing after his death revealed Speck indulging in drugs and sexual activities within the confines of his cell, adding another disturbing chapter to his legacy.

Richard Speck's reign of terror left an indelible impact on the American psyche, reminding society of the lurking dangers embodied by such unpredictable and violent individuals. His story offers no neat conclusions, only a haunting reminder of the complexities within the human mind and the ultimate costs of unchecked rage.

Joachim Kroll

In the shadowy, desolate landscape of 20th-century crime, Joachim Kroll remains a figure of grim fascination. Born in 1933 in the small town of Hindenburg, Germany, his path to becoming one of the country's most notorious serial killers is a troubling study of cumulative psychological and environmental calamity. As the eighth child in a family burdened by poverty, Kroll's early life was rife with hardship and neglect, contributing to a malformed psyche that would manifest in horrifying ways.

Kroll's crimes, which persisted over two decades, were characterized by a barbarity that stunned the investigators who eventually apprehended him. Unlike the methodical Ted Bundy or the notorious Zodiac Killer, Kroll's actions were driven by a grotesque compulsion that combined murder with acts of cannibalism. His modus operandi was chillingly consistent: targeting victims in isolated areas, overpowering them with his brute strength, and leaving a trail of gruesome discoveries for law enforcement to unravel.

In dissecting the mind of Joachim Kroll, psychologists and criminal profilers have often pointed to his intellectual limitations as a significant factor. Considered to have below-average intelligence, Kroll lacked the conventional cunning of some of his contemporaries in crime. Yet, with a predator's instinct, he evaded capture for many years, a testament to the often unpredictable nature of human malevolence. His mental deficiency, however, didn't preclude a sense of cunning: he was known to watch as the police searched for him, reveling in the chaos he caused.

The capture of Kroll in 1976 unveiled a staggering reality; the man known locally as "Uncle Joachim" or "Der Eierdieb" was not just an odd, quiet neighbor, but a monster responsible for at least 14 murders. It was a single plumbing issue that led to his downfall, as neighbors called in technicians for blocked pipes only to find human remains clogging the system. This grotesque revelation unlocked a cascade of confessions from Kroll, each more harrowing than the last, detailing his heinous acts without remorse.

Kroll's trial and subsequent conviction in 1982 marked the end of one of Germany's most sinister chapters. Unlike some infamous killers who sought the limelight, Kroll's demeanor in court was one of detached indifference, as if departing reality altogether. He was sentenced to life imprisonment, a judgment met with relief and horror, serving until his death in 1991. His story serves as a sobering reminder of the depths of human darkness and the challenges faced by those working to understand and prevent such crimes.

The legacy of Joachim Kroll is not merely of the brutality he enacted but of the profound questions he leaves in his wake—about insanity, culpability, and the essence of evil. Understanding Kroll requires a look beyond the mere facts of his crimes, delving into the complexities of a psyche warped by factors both internal and external. His life and acts offer a chilling testament to the need for continued examination of those who dwell on the fringes of humanity, lest they slip through the cracks of societal vigilance.

Charles Starkweather

In the annals of American crime, Charles Starkweather stands out as a symbol of youthful rebellion gone catastrophically wrong. His spree, which left a trail of bloodshed across Nebraska and Wyoming during the winter of 1958, shocked a nation and cemented his place among the infamous killers of the 20th century. Starkweather was only 19 years old when he embarked on this brutal journey, but his actions revealed a capacity for violence that belied his tender age.

Starkweather's story is intertwined with that of his 14-year-old girlfriend, Caril Ann Fugate. Together, they carved a path of death that spread fear across the heartland. While Caril's role in the killings remains a topic of debate, Starkweather's intent was clear. He seemed to be driven by a deep-seated rage and a desire to rebel against the societal norms that he felt had wronged him. This cocktail of youthful defiance and unrestrained aggression resulted in the deaths of 11 people over the course of two months.

Born into a working-class family in Lincoln, Nebraska, Starkweather struggled with a speech impediment and a mild birth defect, both of which made him the target of bullying and ridicule during his formative years. These early experiences contributed to a growing resentment towards society and an emerging fascination with outlaws and anti-heroes. James Dean's portrayal of the troubled teen in "Rebel Without a Cause" resonated deeply with Starkweather, offering a model of rebellion that he aspired to emulate—a dangerous aspiration that foreshadowed his future crimes.

The spree began with the murder of a gas station attendant in Lincoln, an act that would set Starkweather and Fugate on their infamous path. The violence escalated as they fled westward, their crimes growing increasingly brazen and horrifying. Innocent families were slaughtered in their homes, the brutality of the acts shocking even the most seasoned law enforcement officers. Starkweather's cold-blooded killing spree captivated the media, transforming him into a notorious figure and a symbol of mid-20th-century America's fears around teenage delinquency.

Starkweather's eventual capture marked the end of one of the most intense manhunts in American history. His trial was swift and sensational, drawing widespread media attention. Convicted of first-degree murder, he was sentenced to death and executed in the electric chair at the tender age of 20. Caril Ann Fugate was sentenced to life in prison, later paroled after serving 18 years.

Analyzing Starkweather's grim trajectory offers insights into the volatile mix of psychological, social, and environmental factors that can contribute to such acts of violence. While his story is that of a troubled youth driven to extremes, it also serves as a cautionary tale about the potential for latent violence in the seemingly ordinary, prompting reflections on the mechanisms of justice and the societal conditions that can give rise to a killer. Starkweather's dark legacy continues to resonate, providing a chilling case study in the examination of criminal minds.

Ottis Toole and Henry Lee Lucas

Ottis Toole and Henry Lee Lucas occupy a dark, infamous chapter in the chronicles of late 20th-century serial killers. They were a chilling duo, renowned not only for their gruesome crimes but also for the chaotic trail of confessions—and recantations—they left behind. Toole and Lucas's partnership in crime forged a path of terror, characterized by violence, manipulation, and deceit. Both men came from harrowing backgrounds, shaped by instability and abuse, which seemed to pave their way toward a life of crime.

Toole's childhood was marked by neglect and extreme abuse; he claimed sexual abuse by family members and was often mocked for his sexuality. Toole's psychological profile paints the picture of a man deeply troubled and prone to violence. His counterpart, Lucas, had an equally grim upbringing. Lucas experienced brutality at the hands of his mother, who dressed him as a girl and beat him regularly. Such early-life experiences, filled with neglect and cruelty, likely fueled their violent tendencies later in life—a twisted intersection of nurture gone awry.

Their paths crossed in the late 1970s, and together, they embarked on a reign of terror where the lines between fact and fiction often blurred. Lucas's confessions, sometimes staggering in their number and vivid in detail, captivated law enforcement but also cast doubt due to inconsistencies and ever-changing stories. Together, Toole and Lucas claimed responsibility for hundreds of murders, though the veracity of many of these confessions remains suspect. The duo reveled in the notoriety, often relishing the attention they garnered from the media and investigators.

The criminal partnership between Lucas and Toole offers a compelling study into the dynamics between serial killers. Their relationship was convoluted, fraught with manipulations and betrayals. At times, they seemed to fuel each other's darkest impulses, a mutual reinforcement of violence and depravity. However, their alliance also had an element of boastful exaggeration, throwing investigators into a maze of truth, lies, and bluster. This intricate dance of confession and denial made it challenging for law enforcement to decipher the true extent of their crimes.

Ultimately, their separate arrests in the early 1980s brought an end to their violent spree. Lucas was arrested first in 1983, and his confessions to numerous murders initially seemed like a breakthrough. Yet, the veracity of these confessions came under scrutiny, revealing the complexities and pitfalls in relying solely on the word of a notorious liar. Toole, apprehended shortly after Lucas, further muddied the waters with his own conflicting accounts.

The cases of Ottis Toole and Henry Lee Lucas remain emblematic of the challenges faced in criminal justice, particularly the difficulty in handling confessions that are both plentiful and unreliable. Their tales continue to intrigue those interested in true crime and psychology, offering insights into the chaotic minds of killers who thrived on the infamy their horrific deeds brought. In the end, their story serves as a grim reminder of the human capacity for violence and deception, leaving behind a haunting legacy in the annals of crime history.

Chapter 3:
The Psychology Behind
Female Serial Killers

Delving into the minds of female serial killers reveals a complex web of emotional and psychological intricacies distinct from their male counterparts. These women often navigate a tapestry woven with personal vendettas, the pursuit of power, or a distorted sense of justice, transcending mere notions of evil or madness. While men may often kill for thrill or lust, female serial killers typically reflect deeper relational dynamics and motivations. Their killings can stem from a lifetime of brewing grievances, profound psychological trauma, or an acute need for control and manipulation in oppressive environments. Throughout history, these killers were often dismissed as anomalies or overshadowed by infamous male serial killers, yet their crimes demand a unique understanding. By unraveling their psychological motives, we lay bare the societal and personal factors that drive such harrowing acts, offering a sobering glimpse into the darker corners of human nature.

Exploring Aileen Wuornos' Motivations

Aileen Wuornos' story is a tapestry woven with threads of despair, abuse, and societal neglect. She stands out among female serial killers, not merely due to the brutal nature of her crimes but because of the complex psychological landscape that drove her. Understanding Aileen Wuornos involves delving into a life marred by trauma and examining the precarious intersection of victimhood and violence. Her motivations, shrouded in a mixture of survival instincts and fury, compel us to explore the darker recesses of human nature.

Wuornos' early life was far from a nurturing environment. Born in 1956, her childhood was punctuated by abandonment and abuse. Her father, in prison when she was born, later committed suicide. Her mother vanished when Wuornos was just four years old, leaving her and her brother to be raised by grandparents. These weren't warm and supportive guardians; instead, they subjected her to a harsh existence devoid of love and filled with physical and emotional abuse. It was during this time that the seeds of Wuornos' future violence were unknowingly sown.

Her teenage years further mirrored the instability of her childhood. Wuornos was pregnant by 14, and subsequently, she was put up for adoption when her grandmother passed away, and her grandfather kicked her out. Her life spiraled into transient existence, living as an itinerant. She sustained herself through sex work, using her earnings as a means to survive an unforgiving world. This lifestyle was not merely an occupation but a grim reflection of the exploitation she had faced throughout her life.

Many view Wuornos as acting out of rage and desperation. The men she killed differed from typical victims of serial crimes. They weren't targeted for fame or revenge but represented a broader symbol of threat in her life. Society had trained her to see men as oppressors, not protectors. Her murders weren't premeditated in the traditional sense; they were, at least from her perspective, acts of self-preservation. Each trigger pulled, a defense mechanism born out of fear, disillusionment, and deeply ingrained distrust.

The deep-seated anger within Wuornos may be interpreted as a byproduct of repeated victimization. Abuse and abandonment compounded over the years, crystallizing into an explosive form of resentment. Her confessions and trials reveal glimpses of a fractured identity, torn between her hurt and the heinous acts she knew she had committed. Wuornos herself often shifted narratives about her motivations and mental state, at times claiming self-defense and at other times acknowledging the brutality of her actions.

Psychologically, Wuornos challenges the mold of the traditional serial killer. While motives vary widely even within this unique category, many serial killers are driven by sadistic desires or power trips. Wuornos, it seems, was motivated by a convergence of survival instinct, historical trauma, and a profound revulsion for her circumstances. Her actions might be classified outside the standard motive categories of lust, power, thrill, financial gain, or solution to a problem. Instead, they lie at the confluence of fear and anger, perhaps best described as reactionary violence borne out of a tumultuous life.

In dissecting Aileen Wuornos' motivations, one encounters the broader discussion of gender dynamics in serial crimes. Female serial killers often have motivations that starkly contrast with their male counterparts, rarely aligning with the dehumanized portrayals that media sometimes crafts. Unlike the calculated coldness of a Ted Bundy or the manipulative nature of a Charles Manson, Wuornos employed violence not as a means of exerting dominance but, paradoxically, as an attempt to reclaim control over her tumultuous life.

Empathy, however, walks a thin line in Wuornos' case. While her background and circumstances evoke a degree of sympathy, her actions on lonely Florida highways—where many met their demise in her company—are undeniably brutal. The question remains: how much of Wuornos' descent into violence was a product of her environment versus an inherent predisposition to destruction? Her story, though extreme, highlights societal failures to protect its most vulnerable and challenges us to rethink the simplistic binary of victim versus villain.

Media portrayals have further complicated Wuornos' narrative, sometimes casting her as a monstrous anomaly, other times as a tragic figure. Yet, the truth lies somewhere in a murky moral middle ground. Through this lens, Wuornos is both a reflection of an individual psyche and a larger commentary on systemic neglect. Her life and motivations underscore the pivotal role of socio-economic and psychological factors in the development of a criminal identity, challenging us to explore beyond the headline and into the intricate labyrinth of human behavior.

Ultimately, Wuornos' motivations aren't simply about the act of killing but the tragic unfolding of a life scarred by repeated betrayals. Her case beckons us to explore not only what drives a person to commit such acts but also how society might better act to intercept the forces that propel someone toward such a path. Wuornos was a complex character, a woman who, for better or worse, made her mark on history through actions that provoke both horror and contemplation.

Comparing Gender Dynamics in Serial Crimes

When we delve into the psychology behind female serial killers, we encounter a tapestry of gender dynamics that sets them apart from their male counterparts. Historically, society has painted a picture of what a typical serial killer looks like: predominantly male, violent, and driven by savage impulses. Yet, this narrative omits the more clandestine yet equally compelling saga of female serial killers, whose methods and motivations often defy this brutal stereotype. To truly understand these dynamics, it's essential to peel back the layers and examine how societal norms and gender expectations shape the criminal behaviors of women.

Male serial killers are often motivated by a desire for power, sexual gratification, or a compulsion to dominate. In contrast, female serial killers frequently employ the 'caregiver' role as a guise. Those such as nurses or caretakers wield trust as their weapon, exploiting societal assumptions that position women as nurturing and innocent. This guise allows female killers to operate under the radar more effectively, blending into societal norms until their true nature is revealed.

While male serial killers often use direct methods of murder—guns, knives, and strangleholds—female killers typically opt for subtlety. Poisoning emerges as a favored method; it's quiet, leaves little evidence, and preys on the victim's vulnerability over time. This choice is significant and reflects gender-based differences in approaching violence. It also underscores a primal need for control without the physical confrontation that characterizes many male killers.

Furthermore, the victimology between genders diverges notably. Male serial killers frequently prey on strangers, casting a wide net to fulfill their fantasies. Female serial killers often target individuals within their domestic sphere: children, the elderly, or sick individuals. These choices highlight a stark contrast in the relational dynamics that each gender experiences and desires to manipulate. These targets are not random; they're carefully selected and massacred within a narrative of trust and betrayal.

The motives behind female serial crimes also reveal a critical difference. Unlike the frequently sexualized motives of men, many female serial killers are driven by profit, revenge, or a disturbed sense of care. Financial gain, especially within relationships such as familial ties or unjust wills, is a recurring thread. Others may kill out of a delusional belief in mercy or relief from suffering. Such motives add layers to the psychological profile of female killers, inviting deeper analysis of their complex interplay with societal roles.

One cannot discuss gender dynamics in serial crimes without acknowledging the impact of media portrayals and public perception. Sensationalized narratives tend to de-emphasize female serial killers or portray them as outliers of femininity gone wrong. This disparity affects the investigative process, as law enforcement, influenced by gender biases, can often overlook female suspects, slowing down the resolution of cases involving female perpetrators.

Another crucial aspect is the socialization of aggression. Where boys are often conditioned, if not encouraged, to exhibit aggression openly, girls typically learn to navigate their emotional landscapes in secret. This divergence in upbringing often cultivates a facade of outward tranquility, behind which female serial killers hone their lethal instincts. It contributes to understanding why women might commit their crimes differently, harboring violent fantasies they enact in unexpected, covert ways.

The psychological coping mechanisms also vary across genders. Many male killers operate with a tangible detachment from their humanity, exhibiting sociopathic tendencies that numb empathy. Female serial killers often conceal their darkness behind masks of normalcy and emotional adeptness, making their unmasking even more shocking and society's reconciliation with their actions more convoluted.

The societal response to uncovering female serial killers reflects deeply ingrained gender biases. There's often an initial disbelief, a cognitive dissonance, that such evil could lurk beneath a feminine exterior. Case studies reveal how this disbelief can color public sentiment and even legal proceedings, offering insight into the broader societal dynamics at play.

Exploring these dynamics highlights not just differences in methodology and psychology but also the biases and blind spots that have historically hindered a comprehensive understanding of female serial killers. It challenges the prehistoric assumptions around gender and criminality, urging for a reevaluation of gender roles in the context of heinous crimes, and how these assumptions influence both the perpetration and investigation of these crimes.

Chapter 4:
The Role of Nature vs. Nurture

The debate over whether genetic predispositions or environmental influences play a more substantial role in shaping a serial killer's psyche has long intrigued both psychologists and criminologists. As we delve into this discussion, it's evident that the interplay between an individual's biological makeup and their upbringing creates a complex tapestry that is neither easily unraveled nor wholly understood. From the chilling calmness of Ted Bundy to the chaotic brutality of Richard Ramirez, examining their backgrounds provides insights, though not clear-cut answers, to their horrific actions. While some argue that certain gene variants may predispose individuals to aggression, others point to familial neglect, societal pressures, and early childhood trauma as pivotal catalysts. Indeed, the stories of these infamous criminals suggest a potent blend of both nature and nurture at work, challenging the simplistic notion of a singular cause behind their descent into violence. Understanding this intricate dance is essential, not only for unraveling their motives but also in hopes of preventing future tragedies.

Analyzing Environmental Factors

In the debate between nature and nurture, the environment plays a critical role in shaping the trajectory of one's life, particularly when it comes to extreme behaviors, like those exhibited by serial killers. Environmental factors include a broad spectrum of influences, from the family unit to the broader socio-economic conditions surrounding an individual's upbringing. These elements create a tapestry of experiences which, when analyzed, can reveal nuances often overlooked in the pursuit of understanding criminal minds.

The family, often considered the most immediate environment for an individual, sets the initial stage. A tumultuous or abusive family life can sow the seeds of antisocial behavior. Many notorious killers, from Ted Bundy to Aileen Wuornos, reportedly experienced turbulent early years marred by neglect, abuse, or instability. It's not about the occasional misstep by a parent but rather a pervasive atmosphere of dysfunction that can lead to troubling developments in a child's psyche.

Beyond the family, socioeconomic status can drastically affect one's path. Economic hardship isn't an excuse for crime, but growing up in poverty, coupled with limited access to education and healthcare, can exacerbate tendencies toward violence. Children in such environments might witness more crime, turning it into a normalized part of life. Over time, such exposure can alter perceptions of right and wrong, often blurring ethical boundaries in the quest to survive.

The community and culture are the next layers of environmental impact. Communities that suffer from high crime rates or lack cohesive social structures might imbibe a distorted sense of justice or retribution in young minds. In certain neighborhoods, the absence of communal support or positive role models can leave individuals vulnerable to adopting maladaptive behaviors as coping mechanisms.

Isolation plays a more insidious role. Loneliness, whether self-imposed or a result of social rejection, often leads individuals down dark paths. A lack of social ties can foster resentment and bitterness, festering with each real or perceived slight. For individuals like Jeffrey Dahmer, this solitude was palpable, driving urges that culminated in heinous acts.

The weight of traumatic experiences, especially during formative years, cannot be understated. Trauma can manifest in numerous ways, from post-traumatic stress to more insidious disruptions in emotional regulation and interpersonal relationships. Serial killers' backgrounds often reveal a history of such traumas, spotlighting an environment that was less a nurturing ground and more a breeding place for rage and resentment.

Educational institutions and peer groups are environments where future norms and behaviors are shaped. Being bullied or ostracized during school years can breed deep-seated anger and a need for control or revenge. Conversely, those who find acceptance in unhealthy peer groups might adopt negative behaviors to preserve their status, leading down a path of criminality.

The psychological impact of technology and media, particular to recent decades, has become a crucial factor. Exposure to violent media or the anonymity afforded by online interactions can desensitize individuals, impeding empathy and fostering detachment from the consequences of their actions. This environmental shift challenges the boundaries between reality and fantasy, sometimes blurring them perilously for susceptible minds.

Furthermore, societal norms and pressures must be acknowledged. Cultural narratives around masculinity, power, and success can magnify aggressive tendencies in those pre-disposed to them. Society often indirectly teaches individuals what behaviors are rewarded or punished, and these lessons are absorbed, consciously or not, by observing societal reactions to violence and crime.

Ultimately, while genetic predispositions provide a basis for potential behavioral outcomes, it's the environmental factors that nurture these potentials into reality. Analyzing the interplay of these numerous influences offers insights not only into individual cases but also into broader patterns visible across multiple infamous profiles.

The challenge remains to discern which elements within this complex web can be altered to prevent the nurture of future offenders, a pursuit as crucial as it is intricate. By understanding these environmental factors, perhaps society can intervene early enough to encourage a healthier path, breaking cycles of violence before they start.

Genetic Predispositions to Violence

The eternal debate of nature versus nurture in shaping human behavior finds itself at a crossroads when exploring the genetic predispositions to violence. It is here, at the intersection of DNA's double helix and the world's many influences, that we search for clues about the darker corners of the human psyche. Genetic predispositions are not pathways set in stone but rather forks in the road where choice and chance meet nature's blueprint.

Research into the genetic components of violent behavior often leads to discussions around the MAOA gene, popularly known as the "warrior gene." This gene, along with a few others, has been scrutinized for its potential role in predisposing individuals to aggression and antisocial behavior. The existence of such a gene raises provocative questions: Are individuals with this genetic makeup doomed to a path of violence, or is their destiny merely influenced by it?

While genes like MAOA may provide a predisposition, they do not script the play. The environment, personal experiences, and societal influences act as co-authors. A person carrying a genetic predisposition to aggression, when placed in nurturing surroundings, may lead a life devoid of the violence they could have exhibited under different circumstances. It's a narrative that many scientists and psychologists continue to explore with great interest and caution.

The study of twins, especially those separated at birth, offers compelling insights into the genetic underpinnings of violent behavior. When identical twins raised apart exhibit similar violent tendencies, the argument for genetic influence strengthens. However, these studies also reveal the profound impact of environmental shaping, as differences inevitably surface, underscoring the complex interplay between nature and nurture.

Among serial killers, there are often patterns of abuse, neglect, or trauma in early life, suggesting that while genetic predispositions may exist, they likely require certain environmental triggers to be actualized. The notorious killers whose stories populate true crime lore rarely present with a clean slate when it comes to personal histories; rather, their pasts are typically marred by turmoil.

Causal language must be used here to dissect these narratives. The presence of a genetic marker for aggression is not a mandate for violence, yet it may predispose an individual to react more violently under stress or provocation. Here lies the significance of upbringing and early life experiences, painting a broader, more nuanced picture of what might lead someone to commit egregious acts.

In recent years, advances in genetic research have introduced the possibility of predictive analytics, which can identify individuals who might be genetically predisposed to violent behavior. This raises ethical considerations about privacy and the potential for misuse. Balancing these concerns with the benefits of understanding such predispositions is a challenge for modern criminologists and psychologists alike.

Decades of research suggest that genetic predispositions can play a significant role, but they are not deterministic. They can be shaped, molded, and even minimized if the environmental context and personal choices steer the individual down a different path. It is this very interplay that intrigues enthusiasts and professionals in the field of criminal psychology, as it speaks to the potential for both understanding and intervention.

The narrative of genetic predispositions to violence in the context of serial killers requires humility in our understanding. We must acknowledge that while science has made significant strides, many questions remain unanswered. The real-world application of these findings continues to prompt debate, refining our comprehension of what it truly means to be predisposed to violence.

In examining the genetic predispositions to violence, one must remain vigilant about oversimplification. The allure of attributing violence solely to genetic markers can lead us to prematurely label individuals, overshadowing the importance of personal agency and environmental influence. It is within this intricate dance of biology and experience that one's essence is forged, telling a story that is as much about humanity's potential for darkness as it is about the possibility for change.

The intersection of genetic research and criminology is a burgeoning field, with potential applications that could revolutionize crime prevention and rehabilitation strategies. While the path forward is fraught with challenges, the insights gained stand to reshape our understanding of human behavior fundamentally. Those passionate about the dynamics of violence and criminality hold a vested interest in where this research may lead.

Genetic predispositions are a provocative element of the nature versus nurture debate, acting as a reminder of the complexity inherent in human behavior. As we delve deeper into the genetic threads that may weave through the tapestry of violence, we continue to ask the fundamental question: Can understanding these predispositions help us rewrite the stories of those at their mercy, and guide them toward safer, more constructive futures?

Chapter 5:
Techniques of Evasion and Capture

In the murky dance between a killer and the law, evasion tactics and investigative breakthroughs play pivotal roles. Killers, each with their twisted ingenuity, devise complex strategies to elude capture, often manipulating their environments with meticulous precision. Some change identities, others move frequently, or carefully select isolated victims to maintain invisibility. The infamous ones, like Bundy and Ramirez, toyed with authorities through calculated boldness or geographical dexterity. Despite their cunning efforts, the noose of justice tightens persistently, fueled by groundbreaking investigative techniques. Over the decades, law enforcement has evolved from basic fingerprinting to sophisticated DNA analysis and digital tracking. These advances have not only pierced the veil of numerous cold cases but also reshaped how investigations unfold. The relentless pursuit of truth by detectives, armed with ever-advancing tools and methodologies, ultimately breaks the facade of invincibility that even the most diabolical figures attempt to cloak themselves in. By dissecting these cat-and-mouse encounters, we gain profound insights into the relentless drive of both the criminal mind and the tenacity of those committed to bringing them to justice.

Strategies Employed by Killers

Throughout history, serial killers have demonstrated a chilling ability to evade capture, adopting a variety of strategies that allow them to continue their reign of terror. Often, these individuals exhibit a keen understanding of human behavior, manipulation, and deception, using these skills to obscure their activities from law enforcement and the general public. While their motives and methods may vary, a common thread among many is their strategic approach to covering their tracks.

One such strategy is the creation of a double life. Many serial killers present themselves as upstanding citizens, often holding down jobs or maintaining families that serve as perfect covers for their sinister activities. This façade offers them a veil of normalcy that deflects suspicion and allows them to blend seamlessly into society. For instance, Dennis Rader, also known as the BTK killer, managed to avoid detection for decades by appearing as a devoted husband and active church member, even serving as president of his congregation. It was this ability to lead a seemingly ordinary life that allowed him to evade capture for so long.

Another tactic employed by some of the most infamous killers is the selection of victims who are less likely to attract attention. Individuals from marginal or vulnerable communities, such as sex workers or runaways, are often chosen due to their perceived expendability. This grim calculation ensures that the disappearance of a victim might not trigger immediate alarm, giving the killer more time to elude authorities. Gary Ridgway, the Green River Killer, is known to have targeted women in the sex trade, exploiting this very anonymity to continue his spree.

Some killers are meticulous planners, employing careful selection of location and timing to minimize the risk of getting caught. They often operate in areas where they are familiar with the terrain, allowing them to plan escape routes and identify secluded spots for carrying out their crimes. This strategic manipulation of geography is evident in the Zodiac Killer's infamous murders, where the assailant leveraged his knowledge of isolated rural roads to strike and then vanish without a trace.

In addition to selecting specific victims and locations, serial killers may use psychological manipulation to evade capture. Charisma and the ability to gain trust are potent tools that many killers wield effectively. Ted Bundy, for example, famously used his charm and good looks to lure victims. His ability to appear non-threatening made it easier for him to approach potential victims without arousing suspicion, allowing him to strike when least expected.

Moreover, the use of disguises and varying methods of murder to avoid patterns also plays a critical role in evasion strategies. By not sticking to a singular modus operandi, killers can confuse investigators and create disarray. Aileen Wuornos, although not changing her methods frequently, relied heavily on altering her appearance to avoid detection in between her killings. Such adaptations challenge law enforcement to connect the dots between serial crimes.

Some serial killers boast a high level of intelligence and technological acumen, incorporating advanced methods to throw investigators off their trails. Gary Ridgway, for instance, attempted to mislead law enforcement by planting false evidence, including cigarette butts and gum wrappers, at the crime scenes. In the digital age, killers may also employ technology to their advantage, tapping into online forums or utilizing encrypted communication methods to coordinate or brag about their actions anonymously.

Risk assessment is a calculated game for these individuals. Some even inject themselves into the investigation, attending crime scenes, funerals, or police briefings to gather firsthand information that can provide an insight into the progress of the investigation. Such proximity allows them to adapt their behaviors based on the strategies law enforcement might be implementing to catch them. This brazen tactic was seen with the Zodiac Killer, who taunted police and media with letters and cyphers, maintaining psychological control over the narrative.

Finally, there is the chilling strategy of learning from the past. Many contemporary killers study previous serial offenders and their eventual downfalls, carefully analyzing what led to their capture and making modifications to their own behaviors accordingly. This sense of historical awareness, combined with a thirst for notoriety, drives a need to avoid the mistakes of their forebears, enhancing their ability to remain at large.

In summation, the strategies employed by killers to evade capture reveal deep layers of deception, psychological prowess, and adaptability. These strategies showcase not only their cunning but also highlight the ongoing challenge for law enforcement attempting to bring them to justice. Understanding these methods is essential for anticipating their moves and ultimately dismantling the intricate webs woven by these individuals. The convergence of historical precedent, behavioral understanding, and technological innovation continues to shape the evolving tactics of those who dwell within the shadows of crime.

Investigative Breakthroughs

The hunt for a serial killer often hinges on unraveling a labyrinth of deceit, misdirection, and psychological manipulation orchestrated by the killer. Yet, through the veils of obscurity, investigative breakthroughs emerge — not as mere serendipity but through the relentless pursuit of justice. Often, these breakthroughs are the threads that eventually knit together a tapestry of evidence capable of capturing even the most elusive of predators.

In the realm of crime-solving, few tools have revolutionized the process more than forensic science. The advent of DNA profiling in the late 20th century was a watershed moment. This breakthrough technology has led to the closing of cold cases, some decades old, providing answers to grieving families and bringing criminals to justice. The story of how DNA technology led to the capture of the notorious Golden State Killer exemplifies its profound impact. By connecting genetic material from crime scenes with the burgeoning databases of genetic profiles, investigators can now unveil perpetrators who once thought they had outsmarted the law.

However, DNA is not the only weapon in the arsenal of law enforcement. Fingerprint analysis, conducted with modern computational methods, can rapidly match prints across vast datasets, identifying suspects within seconds. In many serial cases, latent prints—once barely perceptible—have surfaced as irrefutable evidence, leaving suspects nowhere to hide. The tenacity of forensic experts can transform minuscule evidence into conclusive proof.

Many would argue that traditional detective work is equally crucial in investigative breakthroughs. This involves piecing together seemingly unrelated events, linking isolated incidents, and creating a composite image of the suspect's behavior. The introduction of criminal profiling, which categorizes killings and predicts future actions, has resolved numerous high-profile cases. By stepping into the shoes of a killer, investigators can anticipate subsequent moves, diminishing the edge the criminal might once have had.

Though technology and methodology are powerful, it is often human intuition that identifies what sheer data points cannot. The nuanced understanding of behavior, developed over countless hours spent examining pattern, motive, and opportunity, allows seasoned detectives to discern the anomalies in a killer's rampage. The insight gleaned from predictably unpredictable actions highlights this delicate interplay between cold technology and warm intuition.

Working patiently behind the scenes, data analysis, and algorithmic models are making significant inroads in predictive policing. Combing large datasets for patterns that evade the human eye is one of the quieter revolutions in crime-solving. These models can forecast where a serial killer might strike next, offering law enforcement a proactive rather than reactive stance. This is a growing field, one that pivots from mere retrospective analysis to real-time action, marking a definitive shift in the law enforcement landscape.

Equally essential are the collaborative efforts between different jurisdictions and international agencies. Serial killers often stretch their deeds across borders, exploiting the gaps in jurisdictional protections and communications. In response, investigative agencies have developed robust frameworks for information sharing. International cooperation has emerged as a critical component, stripping killers of protective geographical cocoons.

A stark example of this cooperation is Interpol's assistance in apprehending individuals who commit crimes globally. These collaborative networks leverage combined technological and human resources to track and capture elusive suspects. Such synergy can dismantle even the most intricately constructed plans of evasion that serial killers devise.

Nonetheless, the breakthroughs aren't limited to technology and international collaboration. The tireless dedication of the investigators can never be overstated. They labor in anonymity, driven not by accolades but by a commitment to resolve the most sinister mysteries. Their pursuit symbolizes the triumph of determination over the malice that lurks in human nature.

As investigative techniques evolve, so does the advice provided to potential victims on identifying predatory patterns or unusual behavioral cues. Increasing public awareness plays a pivotal role in investigative breakthroughs. The eyes and ears of the community, when armed with knowledge, can act as an extended surveillance network, leading to tips, sightings, and ultimately, arrests. Many killers have been caught simply because a neighbor noticed something odd or a passerby were vigilant.

It's vital to understand that while techniques become sharper and more sophisticated, the desire to outwit the law remains ever strong among killers. Investigative breakthroughs demonstrate that this race is not easily won. As cunning and creativity in evasion evolve, so too must the pursuit, each innovation acting as a reminder that every killer leaves a trail, a clue, a fingerprint—a breakthrough waiting to happen.

Ultimately, investigative breakthroughs transform the narrative from a tangled web of confusion to a coherent story with a definitive end. It's a testament to human persistence and ingenuity in pursuit of justice. Each advance ushers in not only new strategies and methodologies but also restores faith in the ability of justice to prevail against the shadows. The relentless quest to outsmart the most twisted minds continues, forging new paths in the study of criminal behavior and ensuring that the darkness that serial killers represent will never go unanswered.

Chapter 6:
Inside the Investigative Mind

Peering into the investigative mind is akin to stepping into a labyrinth of intuition, analysis, and experience. The evolution of criminal profiling has transformed the way detectives unravel the macabre narratives of serial killers, allowing them to piece together veiled identities from a tapestry of crime scenes. Specialists in this field skillfully decipher patterns, motives, and psychological cues that escape the ordinary eye. Through a meticulous examination of the evidence left behind, detectives reconstruct the lives and mental landscapes of their quarry, drawing an unerring line from chaos to comprehension. Case studies of groundbreaking investigations have become chronicles of resilience and ingenuity, capturing moments where a blend of empirical science and gut instinct illuminated the darkest mysteries. The formidable task of stepping into chaotic minds and predicting the unpredictable is no less than a dance on the edge of reason, forever teetering between the known and the unknowable.

Profiling and Its Evolution

Long before the term "criminal profiling" was popularized by television dramas and true crime documentaries, it had its roots in a much simpler form of detective work. Early profiling often relied more on intuition and experience than on structured analysis or scientific methods. In the days of infamous criminals like Jack the Ripper, investigators attempted to deduce the killer's characteristics, though they had little more than witness accounts and rudimentary forensic evidence to go by. Over the decades, however, the approach evolved significantly, transforming into a sophisticated tool that plays a crucial role in modern investigative practices.

The modern concept of profiling took shape largely in the mid-20th century, spearheaded by innovations within the FBI's Behavioral Science Unit. This period marked a shift from instinctual guesses to systematic, methodologically sound practices. Profiling now integrates psychological principles and detailed crime scene analysis, aiming to construct an offender's likely characteristics. Factors such as age, background, psychological state, and possible motives are pieced together like a complex puzzle. The objective is simple: narrow down the suspect pool and guide investigations toward the most probable perpetrator.

Embedded in this transformation has been the significant influence of passionate pioneers. Notably, the tireless work of former FBI agents like John E. Douglas, Robert K. Ressler, and Roy Hazelwood laid the groundwork for contemporary profiling techniques. Through countless interviews with serial offenders, these trailblazers sought to understand the internal workings of criminal minds, eventually publishing their findings to guide future law enforcement efforts. Their combined endeavors crystallized in a more refined strategy that continues to evolve today.

Profiling, as practiced now, is fundamentally built upon the analysis of patterns. Serial offenders often exhibit behaviors that fall into identifiable scripts based on the nature of their crimes. For instance, a killer may consistently target victims of a certain demographic, or leave specific signatures at crime scenes. Such patterns provide the critical insights necessary for building behavioral profiles, which can then be employed to anticipate a perpetrator's next moves. These profiles help guide law enforcement efforts, offering strategic direction in the pursuit of justice.

One of the most significant advancements in profiling has been its integration with other investigative techniques. Before the advent of modern forensic science, many profiles depended heavily on the profiler's psychological and criminological expertise, but modern criminal investigations now benefit from a multidisciplinary approach. Collaborations between profilers, forensic scientists, and data analysts lead to comprehensive investigations that utilize every available resource. The advent of DNA technology and computerized databases has further revolutionized the field, providing undeniable opportunities for cross-referencing profiles with physical evidence.

Despite its advancements, criminal profiling is not without criticisms. Skeptics argue that profiling has yet to fully transition from art to science. While successes are frequently highlighted, there are undeniable instances where preconceived notions have led to erroneous conclusions or misdirections. An overreliance on profiling in some cases can prevent the pursuit of other investigative avenues. Consequently, the role of the profiler is not to dictate solutions but to contribute one piece of a multilayered investigative framework.

Nevertheless, the success stories associated with criminal profiling are difficult to overlook. The apprehension of individuals like Ted Bundy and the Unabomber can, in part, be attributed to effective profiling techniques. Moreover, high-profile cases that have reached a resolution, thanks in part to profiler insights, continue to validate the method's importance in the criminal justice toolkit. Each resolved case offers lessons that feed back into the profiling process, incrementally improving its efficacy.

While traditional profiling focused more on face-to-face interviews and case study analysis, technological advancements have broadened its scope. Today's profilers access global databases and crime reporting tools, layering digital assistance over learned expertise. Machine learning algorithms and predictive analytics are pushing boundaries, offering fresh lenses to review historical data and unearth patterns that might elude even trained experts. These tools don't replace the human element but enhance it, allowing for previously unimagined insights into both historical and active cases.

The evolution of profiling also implicitly challenges societal perceptions of criminals. It prompts an examination not just of crime, but of broader cultural and environmental influences on criminal behavior. As profiling continues to mature, it advocates for a more nuanced understanding of what shapes the criminal mind, considering factors that were previously dismissed or misunderstood.

Ultimately, profiling's evolution reflects the dynamic nature of crime itself—an ever-adapting phenomenon demanding equally adaptable strategies. As new criminal archetypes emerge and behavioral patterns morph in response to societal changes, profiling stands as an indispensable component of investigative methods. It is an evolving dialogue between psychology, law enforcement, and sociology, all intertwined in the pursuit of uncovering and understanding the darkest aspects of human conduct.

In examining the investigative mind, we find that profiling is a testament to human ingenuity in the face of complex challenges. It's a reminder of the endless pursuit for justice, driven by the belief that understanding the minds of history's most elusive criminals can prevent future tragedies.

Case Studies of Notable Investigations

In the labyrinth of criminal investigations, some cases stand out not only for their grisly details but for the unique methods and breakthroughs that brought the perpetrators to justice. These investigations offer a window into the minds of both the investigators and the criminals they pursued, revealing a complex interplay of cunning, innovation, and sometimes sheer luck.

One of the most compelling case studies involves the Zodiac Killer, known for eluding capture while taunting law enforcement with cryptic letters and ciphers. Despite extensive efforts by investigators, the Zodiac Killer remains one of America's most infamous unsolved mysteries. This case highlights the perennial challenges of criminal profiling, forensic limitations of the time, and the psychological cat-and-mouse game between the killer and those hunting him.

Moving from the shadows of California to the world stage, the capture of Pedro Lopez, the "Monster of the Andes," showcases the complexity of international criminal investigations. With over 300 alleged victims across Colombia, Peru, and Ecuador, Lopez's case illustrates the difficulties in tracking a transient killer across borders. It sheds light on how linguistic, cultural, and bureaucratic barriers can hinder the pursuit of justice, and yet how relentless dedication by local law enforcement can eventually lead to arrest.

Another notable case is that of John Wayne Gacy, whose unspeakable crimes unfolded in a quiet Chicago suburb. Gacy's polite and unassuming demeanor masked a horrifying reality, only brought to light through diligent police work and an unexpected tip-off. The investigation demonstrated the power of community vigilance, leading to the discovery of Gacy's sinister secrets buried beneath his own home. This stark contrast between Gacy's public persona and private depravity challenges investigators to look beyond superficial appearances.

Switching from physical evidence to technological advances, the case of Dennis Rader, better known as the BTK Killer, highlights the evolution of forensic technology. Rader's string of brutal murders went unsolved for decades until advancements in DNA analysis and a curious decision to communicate via diskettes became his undoing. This case underscores how patience and technological innovation can converge to crack even the coldest of cases.

The case of David Berkowitz, famously known as the Son of Sam, offers insights into the intersection of media influence and criminal behavior. Berkowitz's spree across New York City turned the bustling metropolis into a city of fear and paranoia. His capture highlighted the roles both public pressure and media frenzy play in accelerating investigative processes. This narrative reflects how modern killers sometimes pursue notoriety, making the detectives' jobs more complex and layered.

When considering legal and investigative breakthroughs, the linked murders by Ottis Toole and Henry Lee Lucas represent a multi-state odyssey in pursuit of truth. Their confessions, recantations, and the challenge of corroborating evidence across jurisdictions encapsulate the often murky water law enforcement navigates in serial murder cases. This case demonstrates the struggles and importance of inter-agency collaboration to piece together the paths of itinerant killers.

Transitioning to the maternity ward, the case of Harold Shipman stands as the chilling narrative of a trusted figure exploiting his power. Shipman, a physician, turned his medical practice into a killing ground, evading suspicion due to his respected status. The investigation that ultimately uncovered his crimes was prompted by a single complaint about an unusual will, leading to the exhumation of numerous bodies. Shipman's case highlights the imperative of vigilance, even toward the most unlikely suspects, and incorporated statistical analysis as a breakthrough technique in clinching convictions.

These case studies emphasize the varied and evolving landscape of criminal investigations, where success often hinges on the fruitful marriage of traditional sleuthing with advancements in technology. The myriad paths converged upon in each case reflect the strategic and psychological acumen required to bring criminals to justice. They remind us that while killers operate from a foundation of darkness and deceit, investigators persist on a journey illuminated by determination and innovation, always in pursuit of truth and justice.

Chapter 7:
Modern Serial Killers and Their Impact

In the tapestry of modern crime, the image of the serial killer looms large, leaving an indelible mark on communities and the collective psyche. From the chilling legacies of individuals like Jeffrey Dahmer, whose infamy extends beyond their grotesque acts to their bizarre hold on the public imagination, to the global reach of crimes that now transcend borders thanks to technology and interconnected societies, modern serial killers compel us to confront uncomfortable truths about humanity. Unlike their predecessors, these contemporary figures often wield the power of media, exploiting a world where news travels faster than ever. This not only multiplies their notoriety but also amplifies the societal impact of their actions, prompting questions about morality, security, and the enduring shadow of fear they cast. As we delve deeper into their twisted narratives, the challenge lies in untangling the complex web of motives, psychology, and impact, while grappling with the implications of a world that both abhors and is fascinated by their presence.

The Notoriety of Jeffrey Dahmer

When discussing modern serial killers, the name Jeffrey Dahmer inevitably rises to the surface, draped in a sinister infamy that both horrifies and fascinates. Known as the "Milwaukee Cannibal," Dahmer's crimes were not just heinous, but bewilderingly calculated.

Emerging during an era when America was already grappling with a series of gruesome serial killings, Dahmer's actions stood out, not because of the scale, but rather the unsettling nature of his violence and his unassuming demeanor in between murders.

Jeffrey Dahmer was responsible for the deaths of 17 young men between 1978 and 1991, crimes characterized by acts of necrophilia and cannibalism. His methodology involved luring his victims to his apartment, under the guise of friendship or monetary incentive, where they were subdued and murdered. This calculated, methodical approach to selecting and killing his victims is what separates Dahmer from many other serial killers, marking him as a figure of profound study for criminologists and psychologists alike.

Despite the brutality of his crimes, Dahmer managed to elude capture for over a decade. His ability to remain undetected for so long can be attributed to his carefully maintained facade of normalcy. Neighbors and acquaintances saw him as a reclusive but otherwise unremarkable individual, further highlighting the dichotomy between his private monstrosities and public persona. This led to a significant impact on societal understanding of what a criminal could look like, shattering stereotypes and inducing widespread paranoia.

Dahmer's eventual capture came about when a potential victim managed to escape, leading police directly to his apartment, where the horrors within were unveiled. The initial disbelief felt by those around him transformed into an overwhelming public obsession once the grisly details emerged. Dissecting Dahmer's life and psyche became a focal point for media coverage, feeding into the growth of true-crime as a genre and altering the landscape of crime reporting.

His trial was a media spectacle. Dahmer's demeanor was disturbingly calm, his soft-spoken manner contrasting sharply against the backdrop of his ghastly confessions. He expressed remorse for his actions but claimed his compulsion was uncontrollable, sparking intense debate over the nature of his mental state. The trial raised probing questions about responsibility, mental health, and the criminal justice system's ability to comprehend and manage such aberrant individuals.

The exploration into Dahmer's psychological makeup revealed a complex interplay of factors that could have contributed to his homicidal spiral. Elements of abandonment, isolation, and burgeoning aberrant fantasies were identified, suggesting both genetic and environmental influences. His case reinforced the necessity for deeper research into the early signs of psychopathy and the role of family dynamics and social environments in shaping potential future offenders.

Jeffrey Dahmer's notoriety continues to have a lasting impact on the field of criminal psychology and law enforcement approaches. The gruesome nature of his acts and his perceived ordinariness prompted a reevaluation of public awareness strategies and criminal profiling techniques. His name has become synonymous with the darkest aspects of human behavior, ensuring his legacy endures as a chilling reminder of the evil humanity is capable of.

The media's portrayal of Dahmer often walks a fine line between informative reporting and sensationalism, a balance which has fueled ongoing discussions about ethical journalism. The public's fascination with Dahmer, while understandable given the uniqueness of his crimes, also poses questions about societal interest in violence and macabre stories. How much this interest influences media practices and justice systems remains a critical area for continued scrutiny.

Ultimately, Jeffrey Dahmer's infamy serves not just as a case study but as a catalyst for change in the understanding and management of serial criminality. His story compels a reexamination of preventative measures, from societal interventions to individual psychological assessments. The imprint of his actions on the collective psyche underscores a reminder that monsters can, and often do, lurk in the least expected places.

The Global Reach of Modern Crimes

In today's interconnected world, the dark shadow of serial crime extends far beyond the borders of any single nation. The arena of modern crimes has shifted, becoming a global phenomenon that challenges conventional perceptions and demands a new lens through which to view them. The spread of information technology and global media has amplified the reach and impact of contemporary serial offenders, allowing their infamy to leap across continents almost instantaneously.

Globalization has facilitated not just the movement of legitimate enterprises and cultures but also of illicit activities, including serial crimes. Offenders today are no longer constrained by geography; rather, they exploit global networks to perpetuate their heinous acts. As societies become increasingly interconnected, so do the criminal paths that these individuals tread. The consequence is a complex web that law enforcement agencies across borders must untangle to bring perpetrators to justice.

The internet has become a double-edged sword in the realm of modern crimes. On one hand, it provides a platform for education and prevention, offering resources for communities to understand and combat criminal behavior. On the other, it serves as a dark alley where modern criminals can hide in plain sight, using digital means to groom victims, distribute illicit content, and trade in illegal goods and services. The anonymity afforded by the web emboldens many perpetrators, offering a perceived shield from law enforcement efforts.

Take for instance the reality of cyberstalking, a form of harassment that transcends geographical frontiers. Stalkers in today's digital age can monitor, harass, and prey on their targets from afar, crossing not just physical borders but the boundaries of personal privacy and safety. As the global digital landscape evolves, the methods by which criminals operate grow increasingly sophisticated, presenting novel challenges to investigators.

Another facet of the global reach of modern crimes is the influence of cultural differences on law enforcement practices. What may be considered an effective investigative strategy in one country might be deemed excessive or even illegal in another. This necessitates international cooperation and the sharing of best practices, although such collaborations are often fraught with geopolitical tensions and disparities in legal frameworks. The urgency of developing unified approaches is palpable in the face of rising international crime rates.

Moreover, the global stage accentuates disparities in resources and capabilities when it comes to tackling serial crime. Developing nations might lack the technology and training necessary for modern investigative techniques, making them more vulnerable to exploitation by sophisticated serial criminals. This imbalance calls for a concerted effort to build capacities and strengthen judicial and investigative institutions across the world.

Modern serial offenders often display an astute awareness of these international dynamics. Some utilize transnational routes and connections to evade police investigations, hopping from one jurisdiction to another, capitalizing on political and bureaucratic loopholes. The ability to manipulate international systems highlights a frightening evolution in their modus operandi and underlines the need for an equally dynamic, adaptable global law enforcement strategy.

In this milieu, the role of international agencies like Interpol becomes critical. Facilitating cross-border information sharing and coordinated operations, such institutions are at the frontier of combating the cross-national spread of serial crimes. However, despite significant advances, challenges remain, especially when it comes to differentiating cultural and socio-economic nuances that affect criminal behavior across regions.

The global reach of modern crimes also extends to the courtroom, where international law must grapple with crimes that break not just laws, but also moral and ethical boundaries. The international legal discourse increasingly recognizes the necessity of bespoke doctrines that account for these crimes' global contexts. For instance, extradition treaties and international courts are called upon more frequently to address perpetrators who evade capture by crossing national borders.

Amidst these complexities, serial crime retains a unifying, albeit sinister, element: its ability to instill fear and fascination worldwide. The international audience following such crimes often fuels sensationalism, perpetuating cycles of fear and intrigue that ripple through societies far from the actual acts. The shared human reaction to these horrific events fosters a global understanding of the profound psychological impacts that such crimes have, both on individuals and communities.

As we delve deeper into the examination of these global dynamics, it becomes evident that combatting the phenomenon of modern serial crime demands not just technology and strategy, but also empathy and understanding. Law enforcement, legal systems, and communities worldwide must collaborate, recognizing that serial crime is not confined by borders nor bound by cultural distinctions. In this collective effort lies the potential for a future where the reach of such crimes is ultimately curtailed, and societies, bolstered by international empathy and cooperation, can confront and overcome the chilling specter of modern serial killers.

Chapter 8:
Media Influence and Public Perception

The intricate dance between media portrayal and public perception becomes even more complex when the subject is serial killers. As news outlets churn out stories of gruesome deeds with sensational headlines, the consuming public finds itself teetering on the edge of fear and fascination. It is a delicate balancing act where the lines blur between information and entertainment, truth and embellishment. In the quest for ratings and readership, media often crafts narratives that can exaggerate or skew realities, potentially influencing collective societal fears and misconceptions. The portrayal of killers can elevate them to almost mythical status, feeding a public appetite for the macabre while inadvertently fostering a cycle of misinformation. This, in turn, impacts law enforcement strategies, public policy, and the justice system as they respond to a society gripped by fear—sometimes more shaped by Hollywood dramatization than by facts. Understanding these dynamics reveals a crucial layer of complexity in the interplay between media and the gruesome intrigues of crime, demanding both critical awareness and responsibility from all media consumers and creators alike.

The Role of Media in Shaping Fear

The media's influence on public perception of crime and fear can't be overstated, particularly when it comes to serial killers. From the grainy newspaper photographs of Jack the Ripper's victims to the 24/7 news coverage of the Zodiac Killer, media organizations have served as both informants and entertainers, crafting narratives as gripping as any thriller novel. This dual purpose—information and entertainment— often leads to a dramatized portrayal of real events, adding layers of mystique and intrigue to the chilling realities of crimes that otherwise might remain under wraps.

The proliferation of crime stories in media originates from a human fascination with the macabre and the unknown. Newspapers, radio, and later television and digital media, have played monumental roles in shaping the collective consciousness and fears of society. As a result, news outlets have consistently dedicated significant airtime and column inches to horrific crimes, not just to inform, but to capitalize on audience engagement. It's this constant loop of coverage that often embeds a sense of fear into the public psyche, making the unknown and little understood aspects of human nature feel present and threatening.

During the 20th century, the reporting around notorious figures like Ted Bundy and Jeffrey Dahmer did more than just describe their heinous acts. It produced an entire cottage industry of serial killer profiling in books, films, and documentaries. Media narratives added layers of speculative personality profiles, psychological analyses, and, at times, even a distorted sense of admiration or celebrity for the killers. Bundy, in particular, was often described in terms that emphasized his intelligence and charm, elements that made him more marketable but equally more terrifying as they reinforced the idea that evil could hide behind a charismatic facade.

The way that media shapes fear can also be seen in the language and imagery it chooses. Terms like "monsters," "beasts," or "psychopaths" are regularly used to describe serial killers, creating a dichotomy of us versus them, humanity against some unrecognizable evil. These descriptors, while accurate in portraying the savagery of their crimes, serve to dehumanize the criminals, almost mythologizing them into figures of horror. This approach not only heightens the drama but also distances them from the reality that they are, indeed, human beings, albeit with significant psychological deviations.

The advent of cable news in the late 20th century and the later explosion of the Internet and social media platforms intensified the media's role in fomenting fear. Now, stories can be replayed, reposted, and shared millions of times, expanding their reach dramatically. The murder sprees of killers such as Richard Ramirez, dubbed the "Night Stalker," capture massive attention partly because they are reported across numerous platforms. This high-profile coverage creates a feedback loop where public anxiety fuels demand for more coverage, which in turn generates more public anxiety.

Moreover, the 24-hour news cycle requires constant content, often resulting in sensationalized reporting. This can lead to public paranoia, as individuals might incorrectly perceive a spike in serial killings, despite false notions mostly stemming from media saturation rather than an actual increase in incidents. The perception of proximity—killers lurking in every shadow—further exacerbates this fear.

The media's influence extends beyond individual narratives to how it frames broader discussions about crime and punishment. For example, news reports often focus on the most gruesome details of crimes, potentially leading to a distorted view of criminality that prioritizes certain narratives over others. These choices can shape public policy and law enforcement strategies, emphasizing punitive rather than rehabilitative measures, under the assumption that severe sanctions are essential to deter what are often perceived as widespread threats.

Yet, the media's portrayal of fear isn't solely negative; it can spark important societal changes. Sensationalized or not, extensive media coverage has, at times, led to a greater allocation of resources to law enforcement agencies and reforms in tracking and capturing criminals. Cases like those of John Wayne Gacy and Charles Manson heightened awareness of the importance of psychological profiling and cooperative efforts between jurisdictions, which have since become standard practices in combating serial crime.

In the modern era, however, the explosion of true crime content—whether podcasts, documentaries, or online forums—has slightly shifted the narrative control away from traditional media outlets. Now, ordinary people, engrossed by crime as a subject, contribute to the storytelling. This democratization of crime storytelling allows for a multitude of perspectives, although it sometimes results in the spread of misinformation or unsubstantiated theories that can needlessly heighten fears and perpetuate myths.

In essence, the role of the media in shaping fear is both a boon and a bane. It serves the crucial role of watchdog and informant, yet often walks a fine line between reporting and inflating public dread. This dual nature necessitates a nuanced understanding from the audience—an awareness that while media can inform and protect, it can equally raise the specter of fear beyond rational proportions, molding public perception in ways that significantly impact societal behavior and attitudes toward justice and morality.

Public Fascination and Misinformation

In the realm of true crime, the public's curiosity about serial killers often strays into the territory of obsession. Stories of heinous acts grip audiences, drawing them into a world that is both terrifying and thrilling. It's a delicate dance between fascination and revulsion, where consumers of media find themselves on the edge of their seats, eager to understand why these individuals commit such appalling crimes. But, inevitably, this morbid curiosity feeds a cycle of misinformation.

The media plays a pivotal role in this cycle, providing stories that shape how the public perceives criminals and their actions. News outlets, television shows, and documentaries craft narratives that can sometimes blur the line between fact and fiction. The details of a case might be sensationalized or oversimplified, leading to misconceptions. After all, the primary goal of media is to capture attention, and in the case of serial killers, nothing seizes it more effectively than a dramatic story.

Take Jeffrey Dahmer, for example. His crimes were so grotesque that they seemed almost fictional to the average person. The media capitalized on this by constantly highlighting the gruesome details, often at the expense of nuanced understanding. This resulted in an almost mythical perception of Dahmer, one that overshadows the complex socio-psychological factors contributing to his behavior. Hence, the public gains a skewed image that emphasizes horror over depth.

Moreover, the fascination with serial killers extends far beyond news stories. It seeps into pop culture, influencing everything from crime novels to blockbuster movies. These elements take artistic liberties, embellishing and dramatizing realities for entertainment's sake. This kind of storytelling further perpetuates myths, like the idea of the "lone wolf" killer, which is far more prevalent in fiction than in real-world scenarios.

Perhaps one of the most insidious forms of misinformation stems from the widespread public platform—social media. Individuals who possess neither the background in criminal psychology nor the investigative insights can freely share their theories and opinions online, often treating speculation as fact. This democratization of voice, while empowering, propagates unverified and sometimes harmful narratives. Depending on the charisma and persuasiveness of the author, such ideas can gain traction, generating a massive echo chamber of half-truths.

The portrayal of killers as either diabolical masterminds or misunderstood antiheroes can distort public perception further. Ted Bundy, with his infamous charm, is often depicted as a "ladies' man," ignoring the heinousness of his actions. Media fascination with his persona sometimes humanizes a killer, overshadowing the brutal nature of his crimes and the suffering of his victims. This misunderstanding glorifies his manipulative capabilities rather than reinforcing the grim reality of his deeds.

Contrarily, when the media fails to understand the intricacies of a criminal mind, it might inaccurately reduce a complex individual to a simple stereotype. Terms like "sociopath" or "psychopath" are thrown around without proper context, contributing to public confusion about mental health and its relationship with crime. This oversimplification marginalizes genuine understanding and discussions about psychological disorders, creating a misleading narrative that they inherently breed violence.

The public's thirst for information often pressures journalists to deliver content without thorough verification, inadvertently contributing to the dissemination of misinformation. In the race to break news first, inaccuracies can slip through the cracks, leaving audiences with edited versions of reality. As stories circulate and evolve, stripped of original context, they can create and reinforce lasting misconceptions.

However, despite these challenges, there's an undeniable responsibility in how we consume and interpret these narratives. Enthusiasts of true crime and psychology must tread carefully between intrigue and scrutiny. To allow genuine interest to overshadow sensationalism, it is essential to critically assess the sources of information and acknowledge when a narrative drifts from documented reality. The truth, while less marketable, holds the key to understanding the minds of history's most infamous killers.

Thus, it becomes crucial to advocate for media literacy. Encourage audiences to question what they consume, seek out well-researched material, and focus on perspectives that offer more than just shock value. Engaging with content through a critical lens helps differentiate between factual accounts and the fiction spun to captivate. In an age where news is abundant and sometimes conflicting, this discernment is more important than ever.

As this book explores the depths of criminal minds, it also seeks to dismantle the myths that have arisen from public fascination. It aims to replace them with a thorough understanding, emphasizing that behind the headlines are human stories of tragedy, loss, and, occasionally, redemption. To unravel the misconceptions, we must look beyond the captivating horrors and examine the systemic failures and societal issues that allow such darkness to flourish.

Misinformation doesn't merely distort our perception of serial killers; it distorts how we perceive safety, justice, and humanity. When we separate fact from fiction, we contribute to a more informed society—one better equipped to confront its fears and bear the weight of its truths. By understanding the true impact of media influence, we can begin to reshape how we view crime and its portrayal in the public psyche.

In the end, fascination with the macabre will likely never fade. However, by embracing the complexities and truths within these stories, we can transform our understanding from superficial intrigue to profound insight, enriching our grasp of human behavior and illuminating the pathways that lead some to choose a life of crime.

Chapter 9:
The Intersection of Mental Illness and Crime

In the murky confluence where mental illness meets criminal behavior, the debate over culpability versus compassion stirs passionately. The tangled web of this intersection challenges our understanding of accountability, urging a delicate balance between humane treatment and the need to safeguard society. Some argue that mental illness can distort reality, leading individuals down a path that defies logic and morality, questioning traditional notions of intent and responsibility. Others contend that the legal system must prioritize societal protection, sometimes necessitating punishment over treatment. The complexity of cases involving mental illness often places them under a harsh spotlight, revealing the cracks in our justice system where legal definitions struggle to match the nuanced realities of psychological disorders. As this chapter unfolds, we'll explore how the justice system grapples with these challenges, searching for solutions that reflect both scientific understanding and ethical integrity.

Debates on Insanity and Accountability

As we delve deeper into the murky intersection of mental illness and crime, one of the most contentious and enduring debates emerges: the question of insanity and accountability. This age-old controversy explores whether or not individuals who commit heinous acts should be held fully accountable if their mental state is compromised. The debate is not just a legal quandary; it's a moral and philosophical conundrum that tests the integrity of our justice system and sheds light on the complexities of the human psyche.

The insanity defense, while rare, is a flashpoint for controversy in numerous criminal cases. Its very essence challenges the core principle of criminal accountability, that individuals have free will and can be held responsible for their actions. However, when mental illness clouds judgment or distorts reality, should the same standards of accountability apply? The courts have grappled with this for centuries, oscillating between compassion and condemnation.

In the United States, the legal standard often revolves around the **M'Naghten Rule**, rooted in a case from the 1840s. The rule states that a defendant may be declared insane if, at the time of the crime, they were unable to understand the nature of their act or distinguish right from wrong. Yet, the application of this rule can be as complex as the human mind itself. Take the case of John Hinckley Jr., who attempted to assassinate President Reagan. His defense claimed he was driven by psychotic delusions. The verdict, finding him not guilty by reason of insanity, sparked outrage and provoked legislative reform efforts aimed at tightening the legal definition of insanity.

Despite public misconceptions, defendants who succeed with an insanity plea don't simply walk free; most are committed to mental health facilities. Yet, the stigma remains—people fear these individuals will re-offend once released. The case of Jeffrey Dahmer, although different as he was found sane, often comes to mind when considering the potential for high-profile offenders to manipulate mental illness claims. His trial, which included testimonies of mental disorders, tested societal thresholds for empathy and accountability.

Aside from legal frameworks, cultural attitudes towards mental illness significantly shape debates on accountability. In some societies, there's a lingering notion that mental illness equates to weakness or moral failing. For instance, acts committed by individuals like Aileen Wuornos are viewed through a lens tinted with gender biases and a misunderstanding of her traumatic history, which played a critical role in her psychological state and subsequent actions.

The narrative is further complicated when considering cases like that of Ed Gein, whose gruesome acts inspired characters such as Norman Bates in fiction. Gein was institutionalized rather than imprisoned due to severe psychological issues. Here, the intersection of mental illness and societal horror leads to an intense public discourse on how best to address criminal behavior that stems from damaged minds, emphasizing whether the focus should be on treatment or punishment.

Psychologists and criminologists also enter this debate by studying the root causes of criminal insanity. Many argue that early intervention in the lives of individuals displaying warning signs of mental instability might prevent criminal acts. However, predicting crime based on mental health forecasts skates perilously close to infringing on personal liberties, echoing dystopian fears of punishing individuals for actions not yet committed.

Moreover, emerging neuroscience research raises profound questions about culpability. If certain behaviors can be traced to brain abnormalities or genetic predispositions, can we hold individuals fully accountable for actions that they may not have had complete control over? This scientific angle adds yet another layer to legal and ethical considerations.

Another intertwined theme is the role of public perception and media narratives. Sensationalized reporting can skew public understanding of mental illness, painting it as synonymous with violence. This misrepresentation fuels stigma, complicating efforts to discern the genuine impact of mental illness on criminal behavior and skewing the legal outcomes of high-profile cases.

The case of Andrea Yates, who drowned her five children, offers another lens. Initially found guilty, her conviction was later overturned due to her severe postpartum psychosis—a decision that brought the nuances of mental health into sharp relief. Public reaction oscillated between sympathy and outrage, highlighting discrepancies in how society perceives maternal crimes when mental illness is involved.

In these debates, the tug-of-war between compassion and justice unfolds within courtroom walls and spills into broader societal conversations. Each case pulls at these lines, redefining them continuously. As society grapples with fair outcomes, the justice system is challenged to find a balance that treats the mentally ill humanely while protecting the victims and larger public interest.

Ultimately, the intersection of insanity and accountability is a dynamic narrative that evolves with every case, historical context, and advancement in psychological understanding. As it stands, the debate remains a pendulum swinging between the scales of justice and the human heart. Its resolution is not only a question of law but one of humanity, threading through moral, ethical, and psychological domains with no easy answers in sight.

Treatment vs. Punishment

At the heart of the criminal justice system lies a profound dilemma: should those who commit crimes receive treatment or punishment? This question becomes particularly knotty when we consider individuals with mental illnesses, especially within the framework of serial crimes. How society answers this question reveals a great deal about its values, priorities, and understanding of human behavior. In attempting to address this issue, we must delve into the complexities of mental health and the limits of our penal system.

Historically, punishment has been the primary response to crime. The justice system, focusing on retribution and deterrence, often dealt with offenders in a manner that emphasized incarceration over rehabilitation. However, psychiatric insights into criminal behavior have gradually influenced this punitive bent, suggesting that certain offenders might benefit more from psychological interventions than from prison sentences. Serial killers diagnosed with mental disorders present a striking case: could a focus on rehabilitation have altered the course of their lives, or even prevented their descent into unimaginable violence?

The argument for treatment hinges on the understanding of mental illness as a significant factor in criminal behavior. Mental health conditions, such as schizophrenia or severe personality disorders, may not cause criminal actions directly but can impair judgment and impulse control. These impairments can lead to actions that the individuals might not have undertaken had they been receiving appropriate care. If society could provide early and continuous mental health intervention for such individuals, we might reduce, if not altogether eliminate, the threat they pose.

Some argue that when crime stems from mental illness, punitive measures alone are insufficient and potentially cruel. The rehabilitation approach contends that treating the underlying psychological issues could not only aid the individual but also enhance public safety. Indeed, many within the mental health advocacy sphere have long called for a more humane, scientifically informed approach to criminal justice, one that recognizes the complexity of the human psyche.

Yet, the notion of treatment over punishment is not without its critics. Skeptics argue that offering psychological treatment to criminal offenders, particularly those guilty of heinous acts, risks undermining justice by failing to hold them adequately accountable. The visceral reaction to crimes, especially those committed with apparent malice and intent, often demands retribution. This perspective sees punishment as a necessary societal mechanism for deterring crime and upholding moral order.

From a legal standpoint, the insanity defense has been a focal point of contention. It raises questions about the extent to which mental illness can absolve individuals of responsibility for their actions. The threshold for such defenses remains high, owing to both legal precedent and public skepticism. Critics fear that emphasizing treatment could open floodgates to abuse, allowing criminals to escape deserved punishment under the guise of mental health issues.

However, the debate extends beyond moral and legal dimensions to practical and policy considerations. Overcrowded prisons and high recidivism rates suggest that the current system of punishment isn't effectively reducing crime or rehabilitating offenders. Incorporating robust mental health services could alleviate some of these systemic issues. Specialized mental health courts, successful in several jurisdictions, exemplify how treatment-focused approaches can complement traditional judicial processes.

The challenge lies in balancing compassion with accountability. How do we ensure that a treatment-based approach doesn't compromise public safety? One solution could involve a hybrid model, integrating mental health treatment with a structured criminal justice framework. Offenders could undergo mandated therapy while still being subject to supervision and restrictions that safeguard the community.

Some cases reflect the intersection of crime and untreated mental illness, epitomizing the urgent need for reform in our practice of justice. While the stories of infamous serial killers often spotlight the depravity of their acts, they can also illuminate systemic failures—missed opportunities for early intervention and support. Examining these can guide the creation of policies that prioritize prevention and understanding over retaliation.

There is no one-size-fits-all answer to the treatment versus punishment debate, especially when it comes to criminal minds saddled with psychological disorders. Each case demands careful assessment, integrating mental health expertise and a nuanced understanding of human behavior. Society's challenge is to craft a justice system that tempers its quest for justice with mercy, one that recognizes the redeemable while safeguarding the innocent.

Ultimately, the tension between treatment and punishment reflects broader societal questions about justice, morality, and our collective responsibility towards those who dwell on the fringes of human behavior. As we proceed in refining our systems, these questions must remain at the forefront of our efforts, reminding us of the complex intersection where crime and mental health meet.

Chapter 10:
Legal Implications and Justice

In the intricate dance between the judicial system and those who have committed heinous acts, justice serves both as a balm to the wounded and a harpoon to the elusive. The legal implications surrounding serial killings are as complex as the minds of the killers themselves, requiring a careful unraveling of motives and actions within the bounds of law. Here, the courtroom becomes a stage where narratives are woven, and the human capacity for empathy is tested against the backdrop of unimaginable cruelty. Notable trials capture public attention, turning courtrooms into arenas of ethical debate and public spectacle. As we navigate the maze of legal definitions and precedents, the boundaries between justice and retribution blur, inviting us to question whether the system delivers closure or merely prolongs the agony of those left behind. Each verdict, delivered with the weight of societal expectation, speaks volumes about the endless pursuit of fairness—a pursuit that attempts to balance the scales for victims and society alike, but also challenges us to reflect on our understanding of justice in the context of profound human darkness.

Examining the Judicial Process

In the murky aftermath of heinous crimes, society clings to the hope of justice served through well-oiled judicial systems. The judicial process, a complex and often harried sequence of events, stands as both a beacon of justice and a source of contention in cases involving serial killers. These trials capture the public's imagination, acting as a stage where law, psychology, and morality collide. How justice is administered, questioned, and perceived amid the chaos paints a vivid portrait of societal values and the essence of justice itself.

At the heart of the judicial process lies the grand jury and subsequent indictment, a preliminary act that can both electrify and polarize the public. For the accused, it's a pivotal juncture. Nothing encapsulates human drama more than the moment when a jury decides whether there's enough evidence to proceed to trial. The criteria for this judgment aren't merely evidence-centric; they are layered with legal complexities and procedural nuances. These early steps often determine the trajectory—how cases are fought or flounder in echoes of ambiguity and uncertainty.

Once in court, the trials of infamous serial killers are not just legal proceedings but public spectacles. They're filled with narratives spun by media, attorneys, and sometimes the killers themselves. Spectators, both in the courtroom and those following through digital or print media, find themselves engulfed in a cauldron of emotions and expectations. The theater of the courtroom becomes a battleground for dramatized truths and bouts of moral reckoning. In every trial, everyone's seeking that singular truth—yet, more often than not, the process fractures it into multiple shards of perception.

The role of the defense attorney and prosecutor cannot be overstated. These legal gladiators strive to outwit each other, one crafting a narrative strong enough to dismantle seemingly insurmountable charges, the other wielding the sword of justice for the victims. Their expertise, or lack thereof, draws lines between acquittal and conviction. In high-profile cases, where public scrutiny is at its peak, the pressure can either hone their skills to near perfection or lead them to critical errors that affect the outcome.

Serial killer trials often bring into focus the contentious interplay between psychiatric evaluation and legal defense. The insanity defense is both a sword and a shield, a double-edged argument dissecting the intricate architecture of a killer's psyche. Determining mental fitness for trial adds another layer of complexity, often involving a dance between scientific understanding and legal definitions. Mental illness and its recognition—or denial—can sway juries, impacting verdicts with a weight that shifts the scales of justice.

The proceedings bring tales of horror and glimpses into the dark recesses of human nature. Jurors, tasked with objectivity, find themselves in a precarious position, balancing their emotions and judgments against the backdrop of presented evidence. They must sift through testimonies, often forced to confront unimaginable acts of violence presented with stark clarity by witnesses, experts, and those who have survived the killer's grasp. It is a heavy burden, and their verdicts echo through history, shaping the narrative of justice and morality.

The media, ever the omniscient narrator, plays a considerable role in influencing public perception. Through every step of the judicial process, the coverage can frame interpretations and incite debates. While it has the power to inform, it equally possesses the potential to mislead—crafting narratives that captivate rather than elucidate. The tension between journalistic responsibility and sensationalism is ever present, affecting the judicial atmosphere and weighing on the scales of justice with an unseen hand.

One can't examine the judicial process without noting the haunting specter of the appeal. For defendants facing the finality of guilty verdicts, the appellate process offers a distant glimmer of hope. This phase usually involves scrutiny beyond the courtroom—the examination of procedural errors or misinterpretations of the law. Appeals drag cases beyond the initial media frenzy but serve as critical components ensuring fairness. They promise that justice, as a system, though flawed, continually strives towards a distant horizon of fairness and truth.

The aftermath of these trials reverberates through societal and legal norms, often prompting legislative reviews and reforms. High-profile cases inspire discussions about penalties, the efficacy of the death penalty versus life imprisonment, and the rehabilitation—or lack thereof—of disturbed individuals. They challenge lawmakers, often resulting in shifts in legal policies aimed at preparing society for potential future horrors.

This section, then, acts as a canvas—painting a picture of the legal gauntlet faced in the pursuit of justice for profound crimes. While it navigates through shadows of the judiciary system, it also sheds light on humanity's undying quest for truth, perpetrating a balancing act between justice, punishment, and understanding.

Notable Trials and Their Outcomes

The courtroom has always served as a stark stage, illuminating the darkest recesses of human nature. In the world of high-profile murder cases, it is here that society grapples with the unfathomable acts committed by those who walk among us. The trials of notorious serial killers offer a lens into these extraordinary events, presenting a mix of legal drama, societal reaction, and psychological analysis.

Ted Bundy, one of the most infamous serial killers, transformed his trial into an unsettling spectacle. Representing himself in court, Bundy's trial in the late 1970s marked a media frenzy unlike any other. His charm contrasted starkly with the brutality of his crimes, creating a public fascination that followed every move he made. Bundy's trial not only exposed the loopholes and challenges in the judicial process but also highlighted the importance of psychological profiling in legal decisions. Despite multiple convictions and Bundy's blatant manipulation attempts, the jury's firm resolve culminated in his execution, a sentence that attempted to close the chapter on his reign of terror.

The trial of Jeffrey Dahmer, the Milwaukee Cannibal, left the world stunned by the detailed confessions of his acts. Dahmer's proceedings in 1992 revolved around the question of his sanity—a recurring debate in many cases involving serial killers. The jury rejected Dahmer's plea of insanity, determining that his calculated methods and concealment efforts pointed to a sound mind. His trial underscored the critical role mental health evaluations play and pushed forward debates about moral culpability and psychiatric disorders in criminal behavior.

John Wayne Gacy, notorious as the "Killer Clown," stood trial in 1980 for the murders of 33 young men and boys. Gacy's trial was a daunting task for any defense team, given the overwhelming evidence—including bodies found beneath his own home. Despite an insanity plea, the prosecution effectively argued his ability to distinguish right from wrong, which led to his conviction on all counts. Gacy's trial is often examined in discussions around how the justice system handles severe mental illness claims, and it increased public understanding of the complexities of criminal insanity defenses.

The mysterious Zodiac Killer, a figure enshrouded in unsolved puzzles, eludes a conventional trial story. Unlike Bundy, Dahmer, and Gacy, the Zodiac Killer's identity remains unknown, challenging the judiciary system at its core. This enduring enigma emphasizes the limitations of the justice system when confronted with confounding cases. The Zodiac Killer's never-ending pursuit serves as a reminder of the importance of adapting forensic and investigative techniques in closing cold cases.

Then there was the trial of Aileen Wuornos, a case that brought attention to the harsh realities faced by women on the margins of society. Wuornos, convicted of murdering several men, used self-defense as her rationale, claiming they had assaulted her while she worked as a prostitute. Wuornos' trial in 1992 stirred debates about gender dynamics, victimization, and mental illness, eventually leading to her execution. Her case remains a controversial example of how justice is dispensed when society's most vulnerable are involved in heinous crimes.

The trial of Richard Ramirez, dubbed "The Night Stalker," captivated America in the mid-1980s. Ramirez's gruesome crimes and his nonchalant demeanor in the courtroom underscored his life of violence and chaos. The jury's deliberation, which resulted in a death sentence, exemplified the notion of a single trial impacting public morale. Though he awaited execution for over two decades, Ramirez's trial remains a reference point for discussions about the death penalty's deterrent effects on violent crimes.

For Harold Shipman, one of history's deadliest medical serial killers, his 2000 trial rocked the United Kingdom. Shipman's breach of trust shook the foundations of the healthcare system as he was found culpable for the murders of over 200 patients. The trial raised questions about the institutional frameworks safeguarding vulnerable individuals and how systemic failures can be exploited by those in positions of power. Shipman's conviction served as a catalyst for sweeping policy changes in medical oversight and patient safety protocols.

The judicial proceedings against Charles Manson, akin to a tragic theatrical production, turned the spotlight on the twisted influence Manson held over his "family." The depraved crimes orchestrated by Manson in the late 1960s demanded public attention as they explored themes of control, manipulation, and societal fractures. The trial's outcome, the death penalty which was later commuted to life imprisonment, reflected evolving attitudes toward capital punishment at the time.

On the international stage, Andrei Chikatilo's trial in Russia during the 1990s highlighted a different bureaucratic backdrop for capturing and prosecuting killers. The Red Ripper's trial, amidst a collapsing Soviet regime, brought long-needed reform to the nation's investigative processes. Chikatilo's conviction and subsequent execution revealed systemic weaknesses but also showcased the growing power of forensic evidence and psychological profiling even amidst institutional turmoil.

In contrast to these historical spectacles, the trial of John Allen Muhammad, one part of the Beltway Sniper duo alongside Lee Boyd Malvo, explored the chilling reality of a coordinated reign of terror. Their trial unfolded in the early 2000s against a backdrop of post-9/11 anxieties. Muhammad was sentenced to death, while Malvo, a minor receiving life imprisonment, invoked broad discussions about juvenile justice and the age of culpability in committing heinous acts.

Fred and Rosemary West, another infamous duo, were tried in Britain in the mid-1990s for a series of heinous murders spanning decades. The Wests' acts unveiled the horrors that could unfurl behind closed doors in seemingly ordinary settings. Rosemary's life sentence (Fred died before trial) maginified the complexities involved in individual culpability versus shared responsibility, especially within criminal partnerships.

Notable Trials and Their Outcomes not only shed light on the mechanisms of justice but also prompt ongoing discussions about morality, humanity, and our ceaseless quest to understand the deranged minds that walk among us. Each trial, with its intricate layers and nuanced proceedings, serves as a stark reminder of the constant interplay between legal frameworks and the depths of human depravity.

Chapter 11:
Prevention and Law
Enforcement Strategies

In the relentless pursuit of justice, law enforcement agencies have adopted a variety of strategies to prevent future atrocities and effectively apprehend those who evade capture. Community awareness initiatives play a vital role, fostering environments where vigilant citizens become the eyes and ears of their neighborhoods, often serving as the first line of defense against potential threats. Meanwhile, advances in tracking and surveillance technologies provide officers with unparalleled tools for monitoring known offenders and piecing together criminal networks with surgical precision. By leveraging both grassroots community engagement and cutting-edge innovations, authorities weave a complex tapestry of prevention. This dual approach not only acts as a deterrent but also as an instrumental force in dismantling the intricacies of serial criminal behaviors, offering a glimmer of hope in the dark corridors of criminal psychology.

Community Awareness Initiatives

As we delve deeper into the realm of crime prevention and law enforcement strategies, one element emerges as crucial: community awareness initiatives. In the fight against serial crimes, these initiatives act as a linchpin, providing both a shield and sword against potential threats. They're designed not just to inform, but to empower communities, making them active participants in their own safety.

Residents who are well-versed in the signs of criminal activity are often the first line of defense, offering valuable insights to law enforcement and providing a network of vigilance that can deter potential offenders.

Community awareness initiatives stem from the understanding that the police cannot be everywhere at once. Therefore, empowering the eyes and ears of the community becomes essential. By organizing neighborhood watch programs and community patrols, residents take an active role in their own safety. These grassroots movements can establish an important rapport with local law enforcement, creating a bridge between civilians and officers that promotes trust and cooperation. Regular community meetings, where police officers, local leaders, and residents gather to discuss concerns and share information, are a vital component of this initiative. Such meetings help demystify the process of law enforcement, reducing fear and suspicion and replacing it with transparency.

The implementation of community education represents another cornerstone of these initiatives. Workshops and seminars that focus on recognizing the signs of criminal behavior and understanding the psychological underpinnings of such acts can be particularly enlightening. By providing educational resources, individuals gain not only knowledge but also the confidence to act on it. For instance, understanding the modus operandi of historical serial offenders—those seemingly small patterns that gave away so many infamous criminals—can help the public spot potential dangers before they escalate.

Social media has revolutionized how communities can stay informed and interconnected. Platforms like Facebook, Twitter, and Instagram serve as digital bulletin boards, offering timely updates on neighborhood activities, alerts, and workshops. They also function as spaces for dialogue, where residents can voice concerns or share experiences. Through these networks, both negative and positive encounters with law enforcement can be showcased, adding a human element to the often abstract concept of policing. Moreover, these platforms can help dispel myths and misinformation that cloud the public's understanding of crime and policing.

Another powerful tool lies in public service campaigns. These campaigns employ various media—television, radio, billboards, and online ads—to disseminate information about crime prevention tactics. The power of repetition ensures that vital messages resonate with a broad audience. Moreover, these campaigns can be tailored to address specific concerns within different communities, ensuring relevance and impact. For instance, a region grappling with home invasions might focus on highlighting the importance of securing entry points, while another facing issues of vandalism might emphasize the benefits of surveillance measures.

Collaboration between schools and local law enforcement also constitutes a vital aspect of community awareness. Schools serve as ideal venues for fostering awareness from an early age. By introducing age-appropriate crime prevention programs and activities, young minds are equipped with the skills needed to navigate the complexities of the world safely. From understanding basic self-defense tactics to recognizing the importance of reporting suspicious behavior, these lessons leave lasting impressions. Moreover, officers visiting schools can break down stereotypes and build positive relationships with the next generation, planting seeds of trust and cooperation that can bloom in the wider community.

On the technological front, innovations like mobile apps enhance community engagement by providing real-time updates and channels for reporting suspicious activities. These apps, often developed in partnership with local law enforcement, empower users to notify each other and law enforcement about incidents quickly and efficiently.

They serve as digital allies, making the sharing of information seamless and immediate, which can be critical in preventing crimes from occurring or escalating.

Engagement with local businesses is another strategic layer in community awareness initiatives. Businesses, through collaborations with law enforcement, can act as informal security networks. Providing training on spotting and reporting suspicious behavior equips employees with skills that benefit not just the business but the larger community. Additionally, businesses often have resources like surveillance cameras that can be pivotal in monitoring criminal activity, contributing to a safer neighborhood.

It's important to note that these efforts aren't one-size-fits-all solutions. Each community, with its unique demographics and challenges, requires tailored approaches. Understanding cultural nuances and socio-economic disparities aids in designing initiatives that are both inclusive and effective. Engaging diverse community leaders in planning and execution ensures that various perspectives are considered and respected.

The success of community awareness initiatives is predicated on sustainability and adaptability. Programs and partnerships should be evaluated regularly to ensure they're meeting their goals. As threats evolve, so too must the strategies employed to counteract them. Community feedback should be sought consistently, allowing for the refinement of initiatives and ensuring they resonate with those they're intended to protect.

Ultimately, community awareness initiatives do far more than deter crime. They knit the social fabric tighter, fostering a collective responsibility that stretches beyond crime prevention. When communities take charge of their own safety, they not only protect themselves but also cultivate environments where trust and resilience can flourish. It's a transformation that's as subtle as it is powerful, echoing the notion that everyone plays a role in shaping the safety and future of their community.

Innovations in Tracking and Surveillance

Technological advances have fundamentally reshaped the landscape of law enforcement and the methods used to track elusive criminals, particularly those involved in serial offenses. As the nature of crime continues to evolve, so too do the tools employed to combat it. These innovations, born out of necessity, serve as both a deterrent and a method of bringing justice long after initial misdeeds have faded into history.

One of the most significant advancements in tracking is the development and deployment of DNA analysis. Initially coming to prominence in the latter part of the 20th century, DNA evidence has become a cornerstone of criminal investigations. This biological fingerprint allows law enforcement to link criminals to their crimes with an unprecedented level of accuracy. The journey from discovery to mainstream integration into law enforcement has been nothing short of revolutionary, and the ability to catalog and compare DNA samples quickly has become an invaluable asset in solving cold cases that had once seemed beyond resolution.

As the digital era enveloped the world, the realm of surveillance saw its own technological renaissance. The advent of digital surveillance systems, enhanced by high-resolution cameras and facial recognition technology, enables rapid identification of suspects in public spaces. These systems, often integrated into urban environments, create a virtual net that empowers law enforcement with real-time tracking capabilities. Such technologies, while occasionally surrounded by debates over privacy, have been instrumental in identifying perpetrators and understanding their movements.

GPS technology provides another layer of surveillance capability that was unthinkable a few decades ago. Not only does it allow for vehicular tracking, but personal devices affixed with such technology give investigators a virtual roadmap of a suspect's whereabouts. The ability to know where a serial offender has been allows for more precise correlations between time, place, and criminal activity, ensuring more efficient use of investigative resources and contributing significantly to patterns and profiles that may emerge.

Moreover, the integration of social media into day-to-day life has offered an unexpected boon to enforcement officials. Criminals often leave digital footprints without realization or forethought, updating statuses, sharing images, and inadvertently revealing locations. Mining social media platforms for investigative leads can corroborate evidence, establish alibis, or, alternatively, dismantle them entirely. The platforms provide law enforcement with a wealth of information that can both solve crimes and prevent future incidents.

While technology undeniably offers profound enhancements to surveillance capabilities, it is crucial to consider the ethical dimensions that accompany such advances. The balance between intrusive surveillance and privacy rights has sparked considerable debate. Law enforcement agencies must navigate this delicate terrain, ensuring that civil liberties are respected while leveraging cutting-edge developments to maintain public safety. Legislators and policymakers are called to establish frameworks that dictate the responsible use of these powerful tools.

Beyond public spaces, technology penetrates private domains too. Digital forensics, a rapidly growing field, delves into data recovery from electronic devices. Investigators can uncover hidden or deleted information, reconstruct sequences of events, and establish timelines with high precision. The meticulous examination of digital traces

114

complements traditional investigative techniques, providing a comprehensive view of a suspect's interactions and intentions.

In parallel, the rise of influence from big data analytics can't be understated. By employing algorithms capable of processing vast quantities of data, law enforcement can predict and prevent potential criminal activity. These systems analyze patterns, flagging anomalies and drawing connections that human analysis might overlook. Predictive policing, while still in its infancy in many regions, promises to revolutionize the approach to crime prevention—shaping enforcement strategies in ways that pre-empt potential dangers.

The fusion of artificial intelligence with surveillance systems propels these capabilities further into the future. AI enhancements enable intelligent video analytics, capable of real-time decision-making without human intervention. Continuous learning algorithms allow these systems to improve over time, distinguishing between routine activities and suspicious behavior, refining their accuracy in suspect identification. Although powerful, the deployment of such technology necessitates strict oversight to ensure data integrity and privacy.

The convergence of these technological advancements illustrates a move toward a more interconnected and intelligent surveillance infrastructure. Each innovation not only strengthens the toolkit available to law enforcement but ensures swifter justice by reducing the time between crime and capture. The speed and efficiency with which modern technology processes information far exceed that of their predecessors, minimizing the risk for perpetrators to evade detection over extended periods.

However, one must remember that no single system or technology serves as a panacea. True success often lies in the integration and collaboration of multiple systems, combining human intuition and technological prowess. Law enforcement agencies world over bear the responsibility to blend these innovations creatively, adapting to the unique challenges presented by each case while staying within legal and ethical boundaries.

Despite impressive strides forward, vigilance remains crucial as developments continue to unfold. Criminals, by nature adaptive and resourceful, will invariably seek new means to exploit weaknesses or gaps in these sophisticated systems. The challenge for those in law enforcement is to anticipate these moves, remaining one step ahead by continued investment in education and technology, ensuring that justice remains served efficiently and ethically.

In sum, the landscape of tracking and surveillance is one that evolves continually, shaped by technological progression and the ceaseless drive of those dedicated to upholding law and order. Innovations in this field not only enhance the ability to apprehend and prosecute criminals but also instill a deterrent effect, sending a clear message to would-be offenders: evading justice is becoming increasingly unthinkable. As this chapter closes, one can only look forward with anticipation to further advancements that will continue to redefine our understanding of crime prevention and resolution.

Chapter 12:
The Future of Criminal Psychology

As we peer into the future of criminal psychology, a fascinating transformation looms on the horizon, driven by advances in technology and a deeper understanding of the human psyche. Predictive analytics, once a figment of science fiction, is now steadily shaping crime prevention strategies by foreseeing potential threats and identifying patterns that may lead to criminal behavior. This predictive shift challenges traditional methods, compelling professionals to balance innovation with ethical considerations. Evolving criminal behavior trends also demand an adaptive response, where psychology intersects with sociology and criminology in novel ways. This confluence aims to not only address the root causes of crime but also curtail its manifestations before they impact society. The psychology of criminals isn't static; it evolves with societal changes, demanding an equally dynamic approach from those who study and combat it. Ultimately, the future holds promise for more integrated and effective interventions that may redefine our approach to justice and prevention, always anchored by the age-old quest to understand why people do the unthinkable.

Predictive Analytics in Crime Prevention

The evolution of criminal psychology brings us to the threshold of an intriguing frontier—predictive analytics in crime prevention. In a world where technology advances at an unprecedented pace, the realm of predictive analytics offers tools for law enforcement to anticipate and possibly curtail criminal activities before they unfold. By delving into vast reservoirs of data and applying sophisticated algorithms, predictive analytics holds the promise of revolutionizing how crimes are understood and prevented.

Imagine a city where police can anticipate likely hotspots of criminal activity not based on intuition or hearsay, but through data-driven insights. This isn't science fiction; this is the cutting-edge application of predictive analytics. By scrutinizing patterns, trends, and correlations over time, law enforcement agencies are now capable of deploying resources more efficiently, potentially preventing crime before it rears its head. Consider the myriad of data that can be harnessed—historical crime rates, socio-economic indicators, environmental factors, and even weather patterns. It's all fodder for algorithms that can help map out the hidden architecture of criminal activity.

The idea of anticipating crime might seem unnervingly akin to Orwellian surveillance, yet it operates on a significantly different premise. While **Big Brother** connotes omnipresence and control, predictive analytics merely offers probabilities, not certainties. Its power lies in its analytical capability to digest and learn from data, rendering a probabilistic map of where and when crimes might occur. Such insights allow police departments to strategize, allocate resources effectively, and enhance preventive measures, thus fostering safer communities.

One of the significant advantages of deploying predictive analytics in law enforcement is its ability to identify potential risks before they metastasize into larger threats. For instance, a notable case involves the Los Angeles Police Department's adoption of location-based predictive policing, which resulted in a 33% decrease in burglaries in some precincts. By utilizing algorithms that factor in data from various sources—like social services or housing authorities—police can generate forecasts about potential hives of criminal activity. This proactive approach signifies a paradigm shift from traditional reactionary methods to more strategic, action-oriented tactics.

Of course, the use of predictive analytics in crime prevention is not without its challenges and criticisms. Concerns about data privacy and the ethical implications of profiling cannot be swept under the rug. Critics argue that reliance on such data could perpetuate existing biases found in law enforcement practices. The question arises—does the data inadvertently highlight certain communities, branding them as inherently more prone to crime? It's imperative to address such concerns to ensure that predictive analytics serves as a tool for justice and equality, rather than a digital enforcer of stereotypes.

Moreover, the success of predictive analytics hinges on the quality and comprehensiveness of the data it analyzes. Incomplete or biased data sets can skew predictions, often leading to misallocations of police resources and potential violations of civil liberties. Maintaining the quality of data, preventing bias, and ensuring transparency in how these tools are used are critical for their ethical application and overall efficacy.

Incorporating insights from multiple domains is another demanding yet rewarding aspect of predictive analytics in crime prevention. Criminal behaviors are multifaceted, often influenced by an amalgam of social, psychological, economic, and environmental factors. Algorithms that analyze crime data must, therefore, be able to adapt and integrate models from diverse disciplines. This synthesis requires collaboration among data scientists, sociologists, psychologists, and law enforcement professionals to develop comprehensive predictive systems.

While predictive analytics provides a formidable tool to anticipate crime trends, coupling it with community engagement initiatives can enhance its effectiveness. Engaging the community in crime prevention strategies ensures that predictive insights are grounded in social realities. It forges a partnership between the police and the community, encouraging shared responsibility in maintaining public safety. Community feedback can also serve as a valuable data source, enriching the analytics with local knowledge and context.

As we stand at this intersection of technology and policing, one cannot ignore the transformative potential that lies within predictive analytics. By harnessing the power of data, we take a significant step towards reinventing law enforcement strategies, not merely as a reaction to crime but as a preemptive measure—a vigilant eye toward a future with fewer victims, fewer crimes, and a safer society. Yet, this future is contingent upon striking a delicate balance between leveraging data and respecting fundamental human rights.

Looking forward, as the tools of predictive analytics continue to evolve and improve, they could potentially reshape the entire landscape of crime prevention. As machine learning and artificial intelligence advance, we might witness even more refined predictive models capable of not just identifying crime-prone locations but also evaluating potential individual behavior based on risk factors. However, with such powerful technology at our disposal, the conversation about ethics and data protection must evolve at a parallel pace. Only then can predictive analytics reach its full potential in preventing crime while safeguarding human rights.

Thus, predictive analytics marks a new era in the future of criminal psychology, encompassing both the promise of enhanced public safety and the challenge of ensuring ethical application. As law enforcement agencies integrate these predictive tools into their operations, they must do so with careful consideration of the ethical implications and a deep commitment to transparency and accountability. The road ahead is promising yet challenging, demanding vigilance and thoughtful discourse to harness predictive analytics in the service of justice and societal well-being.

Evolving Trends in Criminal Behavior

In the constantly shifting landscape of crime, understanding how criminal behavior evolves is crucial for anticipating future threats and developing effective prevention strategies. As the digital world expands, so do the methods criminals employ. This dynamic relationship between technology and criminal activity highlights the continuous adaptation seen in offenders who seek novel ways to exploit vulnerabilities. The intertwining of digital innovation and crime creates a complex web that psychologists and law enforcement must untangle.

The advent of the internet has revolutionized communication, and with it, the methods by which crimes are committed. Cybercrimes have soared as offenders capitalize on anonymity and the vast reach of the digital world. Phishing scams, identity theft, and ransomware are just the tip of the iceberg. These crimes challenge traditional ideas of what constitutes a 'serial killer' or a 'genius hacker,' as they can often involve intricate planning and widespread impact, eerily mirroring traits associated with the most notorious criminals of the past.

As evidenced by recent cases, social media platforms are becoming hunting grounds for those with deviant intentions. The ability to curate false identities and leverage intimate details about victims creates opportunities for predatory behavior. This digital grooming requires a profound understanding of human psychology, as offenders play on individuals' vulnerabilities similar to how historical murderers manipulated their victims' trust. The challenge for today's criminal psychologist lies in deciphering these new layers of deceit.

Moreover, global connectivity facilitates transnational crimes, blurring the lines of jurisdiction and complicating legal proceedings.

Traffickers and cartels exploit these international channels, broadening their reach and fortifying their operations with logistical support that was unimaginable in the past. This globalization of crime poses new challenges for authorities who must collaborate across borders—requiring advanced profiling techniques and multinational cooperation—to dismantle sophisticated networks.

The use of technology in crimes, both as a tool and a target, prompts a deeper examination of motivations behind criminal acts. In some instances, tech-savvy offenders aren't driven by the same primal instincts that propelled past killers. Instead, they are motivated by the potential for notoriety, financial gain, or ideological spread—distinctions that redefine traditional criminal typologies. Psychologists must reconceptualize why these crimes are committed, considering motives that fall outside the typical purview of greed or impulse.

Artificial intelligence (AI) and machine learning represent another frontier both in the perpetration and prevention of crime. Criminals utilizing AI can automate tasks traditionally done manually, increasing the efficiency and scale of their operations. On the flip side, law enforcement arms itself with the same technology to predict and pre-empt criminal activities. These AI-driven models analyze behavioral patterns to develop probable profiles, giving authorities a proactive edge but also raising ethical concerns about privacy and presumption.

Underground forums and encrypted networks like the dark web offer sanctuaries for illicit trade and communication. These hidden realms provide anonymity and discretion, emboldening participants to engage in illegal activities without fear of exposure. From narcotics and firearms to trafficking in human lives, the dark web exacerbates issues surrounding accountability and enforcement. This insidious market demands innovative solutions that balance surveillance with civil liberties—no small feat for contemporary justice systems.

Financial crime is another arena adapting rapidly alongside evolving criminal behavior. Cryptocurrencies and blockchain technology, initially lauded for their potential in decentralizing finance, also provide near-untraceable channels for money laundering and fraud. The intersection of financial crime with traditional criminal enterprises exemplifies the adaptability of criminals who continuously adjust tactics to stay ahead of enforcement. The sophistication of these operations demands a multi-disciplinary approach, integrating insights from psychology, criminology, and digital forensics.

On a more local level, the rise of personalized medicine and genetic editing opens uncomfortable avenues for exploitation. The illegal market for genetic data and biotechnology products places a premium on biometric security and privacy, making individuals vulnerable to identity theft at the genomic level. The potential misuse of genetic information for nefarious purposes, such as targeted bioweapons or espionage, adds yet another layer of complexity to modern criminal psychology.

In tandem with these technological developments, sociopolitical trends impact criminal behavior. Economic disparities, political unrest, and cultural upheavals contribute to an ecosystem where crime thrives. Desperation and disenfranchisement often lead to radicalization and extremism, feeding into narratives that justify heinous acts. This socio-psychological interplay must be scrutinized to dismantle the roots of criminal behavior in an increasingly polarized world.

Finally, the psychological profile of modern criminals is ever-evolving. While some trends mirror those of historic figures, today's offenders might not fit neatly into established categories. There's an increasing need for criminal psychologists to adapt and refine their models to factor in new motivations and opportunities. By grasping these evolving trends, society can better prepare for an uncertain future where criminal psychology must continually adapt to meet emerging challenges.

As we cast our gaze forward, the urgency to understand these evolving trends in criminal behavior grows. With each new technological advance, there is potential for both constructive and destructive use. By staying ahead of the curve, society can not only anticipate criminal innovations but also fortify the means to counteract them. Through concerted efforts, an evolving understanding of criminal psychology can be both our shield and our lens into a safer tomorrow.

Conclusion

In the intricate tapestry of crime, the figures that stand out most starkly are those who defy the very fabric of human empathy and morality—serial killers. As we've journeyed through this exploration of infamous individuals who have committed heinous acts, we've seen how each killer's motives, methods, and psychological profiles reflect broader questions about the human condition. Serial killers are not mere anomalies in society; they are products of specific circumstances, nested within layers of psychological, social, and biological threads.

Our examination has taken us through the dark corridors of criminal minds, unveiling the key influences that contribute to the making of a killer. Followers of this narrative have tapped into a critical understanding that early childhood experiences, often laced with trauma or neglect, can sow the seeds for future violence. The intersection of nature and nurture remains a focal point of discussion, shedding light on how genetic predispositions paired with a tumultuous environment craft the minds of these notorious figures.

The riveting tales of Ted Bundy, Jeffrey Dahmer, and others cast a shadow large enough to be remembered across generations. These stories, although chilling, underscore a significant dissonance between an individual's public persona and their hidden, violent selves. We recognize in these stories not merely a fascination with evil but a means to make sense of the aberrations within human conduct. It challenges us to consider how monsters are made and how they roam among us, often undetected until it's too late.

It becomes apparent that understanding the psychological profiles of these killers can serve not just as a means of demystifying their actions but as a blueprint for preventing future tragedies. Our exploration into female serial killers, such as Aileen Wuornos, further emphasizes that serial murder is not a monolith; it's a complex tapestry that necessitates varied perspectives, including the lens of gender dynamics. Female serial killers often exhibit different motivations, which are essential in enriching our understanding of this criminal phenomenon.

The methodologies employed by law enforcement to track down these individuals have evolved remarkably over time. Through the advancement of investigative techniques and strategic profiling, authorities have cracked cases that previously baffled entire communities. Each solved case is a testament to human ingenuity and determination. The media, while a powerful tool in bringing these stories to the public, often wields a dual-edged sword; it shapes fear but can also mislead through sensationalism, further complicating public perception of these criminals.

With modern technology and data analytics, we stand on the cusp of a new era in criminal psychology and law enforcement. The integration of predictive analytics offers promising avenues for preventing crime before it happens, potentially saving countless lives. However, this also raises ethical debates about privacy and the possibility of erroneously targeting innocent individuals. The future of crime prevention will undoubtedly balance innovation with responsibility.

Within the realms of mental illness and crime, the line between insanity and accountability remains contentious. Arguments rage on regarding the appropriateness of punishment versus treatment in cases involving serial killers. The justice system continuously grapples with these questions, aiming to deliver fair trials and just outcomes. Notable cases often set benchmarks for legal discourse and reform, posing questions about how societies choose to enact justice.

Ultimately, as we look ahead, the prevention of serial crime rests significantly on community awareness and proactive law enforcement strategies. Educating the public, coupled with leveraging technological innovations, holds the potential to curb future threats. Each community's vigilance plays a pivotal role in creating a safer environment, where the realization of such tragedies becomes increasingly rare.

This exploration does not conclude with simple answers; rather, it invites ongoing dialogue and inquiry. Serial killers serve as a reminder of humanity's darkest potential but also our capacity for understanding and counteraction. As a society armed with knowledge, compassion, and a relentless quest for justice, we inch closer to a future where these dark figures are merely relics of the past, obliterated by the light of human progress. Through continued study, collaboration, and compassion, we pave the path towards a safer and more enlightened world.

www.ingramcontent.com/pod-product-compliance
Lightning Source LLC
Chambersburg PA
CBHW040952170526
45159CB00013B/3109